BIG BIG LOVE

BIG BIG LOVE

A Sex and
Relationships Guide
for People of Size
(and Those Who
Love Them)

Hanne Blank

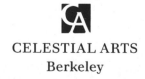

CELESTIAL ARTS
Berkeley

Text copyright © 2000, 2011 by Hanne Blank
Illustrations copyright © 2011 by Elizabeth Tamny
Front cover photograph copyright © 2011 by Molly Bennett/Fat Bottom Boudior

All rights reserved.
Published in the United States by Celestial Arts, an imprint of the
Crown Publishing Group, a division of Random House, Inc., New York.
www.crownpublishing.com
www.tenspeed.com

Celestial Arts and the Celestial Arts colophon are registered trademarks
of Random House, Inc.

A previous edition of this work was published in the United States by
Greenery Press, Gardena, California, in 2000.

Library of Congress Cataloging-in-Publication Data
Blank, Hanne.
  Big big love : a sex and relationship guide for people of size
(and those who love them) / by Hanne Blank. — Rev. ed.
      p. cm.
  Includes index.
  Summary: "A comprehensive and practical guide on the how-tos and
why-tos of love, romance, and great big sexuality for everyone—regardless
of gender or orientation—from the chubby to the supersized"
—Provided by publisher.
  1. Sex. 2. Sex instruction. 3. Sexual health. I. Title.
  HQ21.B64 2011
  813'.54—dc22
                          2011009409

ISBN 978-1-58761-085-1

Printed in the United States of America

Design by Chloe Rawlins

10 9 8 7 6 5 4 3 2 1

First Revised Edition

In memoriam

Heather "Reva Lucian" MacAllister

1968–2007

Fat-bottomed girls, you make the rockin' world go 'round.

—QUEEN

Contents

Preface

Big Big Love **had its beginnings** in a 'zine I did with my friend, illustrator Liz Tamny, in the 1990s. Back in the days when this thing called "desktop publishing" was new and shiny, *Zaftig!* was an attempt to produce a publication focused on fat sexuality that I myself actually wanted to read. I had seen the sketchy, low-budget porn mags produced for straight guys who liked fat chicks. But they were, in a word, depressing. I didn't want pictures of fat women in bad makeup, poor lighting, and cheap, unpretty lingerie. I wanted images and words about people being sexual on their own terms, hot and complicated, not merely offering themselves up, with a whiff of hope-against-hope, to maybe just this once be the object of someone's desire.

What I wanted was something that reflected my life and my friends' lives. It struck me as a problem that, despite the immense quantities of porn out there in the world, there was really nowhere to encounter the desires and the sexual experiences of fat people themselves, male and female, straight and queer, different skin colors and backgrounds, kinky and vanilla, able-bodied and not—the whole funky mixed bag of fat humanity. Based on the idea that nobody should be deprived of their own image, *Zaftig!* tried to provide some of those images, reflecting some of the many bodies and sexualities that never seemed to make it into the frames and pages of mainstream sexual materials.

Zaftig! didn't last long, even with Liz's valiant work in the design department. I was in grad school at the time and producing 'zines is time consuming. It did, though, ultimately lead to my teaching some classes on sex and sexuality for fat folks at places like Boston's feminist sex toy store Grand Opening!, and that in turn led to my being asked to write the first version of *Big Big Love: A Sourcebook on Sex for People of Size and Those Who Love Them* for Greenery Press. I had never written a book before and had never really given it any thought. Still, I believe, as the British composer Arnold Bax once said in *Farewell, My Youth*, "you should make a point of trying every experience once, excepting incest and folk dancing," so I said I'd do it. I wrote the original *Big Big Love* in a wild flurry, and in February 2000, it was published.

Having *Big Big Love* out in the world was a fascinating and weird experience. It certainly wasn't anything I'd ever expected I'd be doing with myself professionally—I'm trained as a classical musician and as a historian. It was, however, a great learning experience and, for the most part, a lot of fun. I did a bunch of readings and workshops and met hundreds of fantastic, sexy, funny, smart people of all sizes and shapes. I gave a lot of interviews, including to interviewers who were, let us say, not always able to bring themselves to think kindly on the idea of this particular book. I spoke at some conferences, I lectured on some campuses, and I answered a metric ton of email from readers, much of which floored me with its candidness. If I had ever doubted that there was a need for fat people to have their own images reflected back to them in media that celebrated them as vital and vibrant and valid sexual beings, those emails made it crystal clear. Even now I still get reader mail from people who are just encountering the 2000 edition of *Big Big Love*. In 2001, I edited an anthology of fat-related erotica, a companion volume to

Big Big Love if you will, named after my dearly departed 'zine. *Zaftig: Well Rounded Erotica* was published by Cleis Press.

By and by, I moved on to other projects, and eventually the original version of *Big Big Love* went out of print. By that time it was becoming outdated, and, although I certainly had mixed feelings about it no longer being available, I figured it was probably for the best. Then in 2010, Ten Speed Press approached me about doing a new *Big Big Love*, the book you are now holding in your hands.

Although the new *Big Big Love* resembles the original in some ways, and some of the section titles have stayed the same, the content is all fresh and newly written from the ground up. Only the positive attitude, and the general feeling that fat people are sexy people with no need whatsoever to apologize for their bodies, have been recycled. Additionally, thanks to the fantastic people at Ten Speed Press and our delicious, fat-positive, sexy-minded artists, photographer Molly Bennett and illustrator Elizabeth Tamny, this edition has artwork, something the original *Big Big Love* was unable to accommodate.

In putting together this new, updated, and hopefully even more useful *Big Big Love*, I was supported by many, many people in many wonderful ways. My gratitude, then, goes to Sheila Addison, Austin J. Austin, S. Bear Bergman, Will Byam, Leigh Ann Craig, Debbie Notkin, Jenny Erhardt, Anne Gwin, Zak Hubbard, Laura Waters Jackson, Substantia Jones, Kathleen Kennedy, Lesley Kinzel, Marissa Lingen, Keridwen Luis, Deb Malkin, Jude McLaughlin, Lisa Nichols, Golda Poretsky, Moira Russell, Sandy Ryan, Jeannette Smyth, Ned Sonntag, Mary Sykes, Elizabeth Tamny, Cheryl Wade, j wallace, Rhetta Wiley, Liza Wirtz, and Yohannon, along with numerous others. Thanks are also due to interns Kelly Morris and Arianna Iliff, Lisa Westmoreland and Julie Bennett at Ten Speed Press, and the unimprovable Christopher Schelling. To them, and to the Weinberg YMCA on 33rd Street here in Baltimore, Maryland, I owe a great deal of what passes for my sanity. Finally, my profound gratitude goes to Malcolm Gin, my partner of the past fifteen years. Thank you for being my love, my friend, and my favorite coconspirator ever. I really am the luckiest girl in the world.

I am also grateful to every one of the seven-hundred-plus people who took the Big Big Love 2010 Survey, which has influenced virtually every page of this book, and to the numerous anonymous volunteer interviewees whose words grace these pages even though their names do not. Throughout this book, you will find anonymous quoted remarks and insights, set off in a different font, from a variety of self-identified fat people and people who are attracted to fat partners. These quotations come from this one-of-a-kind survey that was conducted specifically for this book. The survey was conducted online, during the months of July and August 2010, and ultimately generated 748 completed surveys. Survey respondents were recruited online, primarily through word of mouth. This is, obviously, not a scientific or a randomized survey, and I make no claims that it delivers an accurate statistical portrayal of the fat population. It does, however, provide representative and often insightful information about the personal sexual experiences of at least a small subset of what is a monumentally large and diverse population of people.

The respondents to the survey ran the full gamut of sizes and sexualities, ages and backgrounds. The average age of the respondents was 34.5 years, but the range of ages spanned from 18 to 73. They were split approximately equally between heterosexually identified, homosexually identified, and bisexually identified individuals (multiple answers were allowed).

Respondents reported that they had made their sexual debut, on average, at the age of 17, and at the time of the survey, the average respondent had had 25.5 sexual partners. "Sexual activity" was self-defined, since not all people choose to engage in the same kinds of sex.

Those surveyed described their own bodies diversely, as "average" (10.3%), "overweight" (29.8%), "fat" (58%), "obese" (14.3%), "thin" (2.7%), and "supersized" (5.1%), and with other terms like "fluffy," "deathfat," "voluptuous," "thick," "chubby," "chunky," "bear," and "lush." They described the kinds of body types to which they were attracted with similar diversity: 94% of them said they were attracted to "very thin" partners, 47.8% to "thin," 88.2% to "average" body types, 67.9% to "overweight" partners, 58.7% to "fat" partners, 22.9% to "obese" partners, and 15.4% to "supersized" partners (multiple answers were permitted). In addition, 94% of respondents said that they had been sexually or romantically interested in a fat partner, while 6% said they had not. However, only 16% said that they were specifically attracted by fatness, while 84% were not specifically attracted by fatness.

On the whole, the survey respondents indicated that, at least among those taking the survey, a robust sexual existence and fatness are not at all a contradiction in terms. In fact, it seems that in this respect as in so many others, it's normal to be normal. Fat people's sexual lives seem to be just as vibrant and variable as they are for any other group.

A Brief Introduction, with a Side of Debunking

Fat people have sex. Sweet, tender, luscious sex. Sweaty, feral, sheet-ripping sex. Shivery, jiggly, gasping sex. Sentimental, slow, face-cradling sex. Even as you read these words, there are fat people out there somewhere joyously getting their freak on. Not only that, but fat people are falling in love, having hookups, being crushed-out, putting on sexy lingerie, being the objects of other people's lust, flirting, primping before hot dates, melting a little as they read romantic notes from their sweeties, seducing and being seduced, and having shuddering, toe-curling orgasms that are as big as they are.

It's only natural. Sexuality is part of the birthright that comes with having a body, just like sleeping and eating and breathing and stretching and wriggling with pleasure when someone scratches your back just right. After all, body size has nothing to do with whether or not it feels good to have that spot right between your shoulder blades scratched, and a good night's sleep leaves you feeling restored no matter what number comes up when you step on the scale. Sex is not so different. We are physical animals, and sexuality is part of that. We're only human.

Not only are we human, but we are legion. Technically speaking, about one-third of adult Americans are obese by the BMI-happy standards of the Centers for Disease Control. At a rough estimate, that's about a hundred million people. Sure, this represents a wide range of people, from folks with a couple handfuls of extra junk in the trunk to the fattest among us, and it represents a wide range of experience. But the simple fact is that, wherever you have a hundred million people, there's probably going to be a whole lot of sex happening, too.

Those are the facts. It doesn't matter how much people love to tell us that fat people aren't sexy or sexual. It doesn't matter that the media—including most mainstream pornography sources—do their best to write fat people's sexuality completely out of the picture, as if it'll go away if we just don't show pictures of it. A hundred million people don't automatically become celibate just because their BMIs drift higher than thirty. That's the bottom line. Fat people having a sexy time isn't just a good idea: it's flesh and blood everyday reality.

At the same time, sex can be complicated and difficult, a source of worry and shame, vulnerability and pressure. So can fatness. Sex and fatness have a lot in common, actually. Aside from the fact that you're not supposed to have too much of either one—and if you do, you're not supposed to admit it or, God forbid, enjoy it—they also both have a lot to do with appetites and desires, the body and our relationships to it, and our deep-seated emotional desires for acceptance and love. Put sex and fatness together, and it can open up what seems like a bottomless pit of issues.

That's why this book exists. Like other people who don't fit into the mainstream model of what is sexy or sexually desirable, fat people have their own particular set of issues surrounding sex. So do the people who tend to desire fat partners or who have, as so many people do, simply fallen in love with someone who happens to be fat. Some of the issues are the practical nuts-and-bolts of sexual activity: Is it safe for a fat woman to get on top? (Yes!) How can you do it doggy style and still keep weight off your bad knees? (Read and learn, Grasshopper.) What if you need a good comeback to some jerkola comment? (We've got those, too.) Of course, emotions come into play, too. Confidence, self-esteem, general self-acceptance, and accepting yourself as a sexual being are complicated for everyone, but they are all the more so when you live in a culture that tells you that none of those things should be possible for you because you're fat.

This is not so much the kind of sex book that will offer you "Twenty-Five Top Tips to Make Her Orgasm Every Time" or "The Six Sex Moves No Man Can Resist." Other sex books can fill you in on practical details, like X-marks-the-spot maps to the clitoris, step-by-step instructions to giving the world's best hand job, and how to outfit an entire dungeon at IKEA. The Resource Guide at the end of the book has a hand-picked list of these kinds of things, all chosen with fat loving care.

What this sex book offers is something the others cannot: it understands from the inside the sexual issues that come up that are specific to being fat. The author of this book is fat, and the many different voices you will hear commenting throughout these pages—taken from interviews and a survey specifically conducted for this book—are all from fat people and from people who prefer fat partners. We've been there. We get it. We know. And when we say that it's possible for a fat person's love and sex life to be completely freaking fantastic, we ain't just whistlin' Dixie.

On that note, an aside about the f-word. Throughout this book, the word *fat* is used in preference to the usual collection of euphemisms. It may be a little jarring at first—in our fat-hating culture it can be more shocking to hear someone use the word *fat* than it is to hear them drop the other f-bomb. But both words are perfectly useful Anglo-Saxon monosyllables. *Fat* is just a word, and a simple, accurate word at that. Unlike *overweight*, it doesn't imply that there is only one weight that is right. Unlike *obesity*, it isn't a medical term with particular implications about illness and disease. *Fat* is just fat, like *bald* is bald, *short* is short, and *green eyed* is green eyed. It just is what it is. And that's okay.

That being said, not all fatness is alike. The degree to which different people are fat varies, and so do body shapes. The way fatness is perceived also varies from person to person and context to context. What would count as alarmingly fat in one subculture might be considered merely thick and luscious in another. Fat women are often not viewed in the same light as fat men. People end up with different baggage about fatness because of their ethnicity, their skin color, their sexual orientation, and their socioeconomic class. No one book could possibly reflect the full diversity of fat people's lives, not even in a single arena. In acknowledging this, I apologize in advance if your specific experience with fat and sex is not mirrored in these pages. Unfortunately, there is no way everyone's can be. Nevertheless, a lot of us do share experiences, and there are lots of things we can learn from other people's perceptions, insights, and lives. Above and beyond that, there is the desire that so many of us share—the desire for more fulfilling, more pleasurable, and more joy-filled sex lives, no matter what size, shape, or weight we are.

To which I say: make it so! And to help you do it, we can start by debunking some of the old wives' tales, urban legends, tall tales, and just plain old lies that our fat-hating culture loves to toss around about sex and fatness. Arm yourself against the misinformation and the lies with this roundup of common fat sexuality myths.

Myth:
No one is attracted to fat people.

Busted! Wrong, wrong, wrong, and wrong. It's actually pretty common to be attracted to fat people. Or to be attracted to people, who come in many different appealing shapes and sizes. It is in fact pretty much universal to be attracted to people whose bodies may change, because change is one of the things bodies

"All of that wonderful soft fat provides the best sexual playground in the world."

just *do*. Fat is one of the things bodies can be. If you are capable of becoming attracted to a person, it is possible that you might become attracted to a fat person.

Some people are attracted to fatness itself and would be categorically turned off by anyone who wasn't fat. Other people are capable of being attracted to a wide range of physical shapes and sizes and may, from time to time, find themselves being attracted to fat partners. It's not uncommon for thinner people to get into relationships, gain weight as time goes by, and still find each other sexy. Many people get interested in someone for reasons having little to do with looks, size, or shape, only to discover—possibly to their consternation, but also perhaps to their delight—that they are attracted by physical qualities they had simply never considered before. There are many different ways in which someone can become attracted to a fat partner.

Size itself can be a turn-on. Just as some people are turned on by very petite bodies—they like the look and feel of smallness—there are people who are turned on by bigness. Some people find it sexy and fulfilling to feel like their partner is bigger than they are. It might have overtones of being overpowered or of being encompassed and engulfed. Or maybe they just like the idea of having all that flesh to caress and explore and revel in.

Some love the look of big bodies. The slopes and curves of fat bodies are luxurious. They can give a sense of durability, of permanence, of power, of comfort and abundance. Fatness can also magnify gender. For some people, fat makes secondary sexual characteristics more pronounced. Many fat men look solid and heavy through the torso, thick and burly. Many fat women have sumptuous curves and cleavage for days. Depending on how they are shaped,

> "Fat feels absolutely incredible, looks incredible too. Nothing else gets me nearly as turned on. Rounded facial features add an element of cuteness, while the large breasts, legs and thighs, and butt are overwhelmingly hot and sexy. I love the feeling of the entire body, either during foreplay, sex, or cuddling. I love going down on a nice fat mons pubis with nice plush lips to suck on."

and where their bodies tend to carry fat, fat people's bodies can evoke idealized and intense masculinity or femininity. Or, again depending on how one is shaped, the gender magnification can go the other way, creating an enticing sense of androgyny or genderfuck. (I've noticed many sexy fat butches and transmasculine people using this to their advantage.)

"I like female or trans-identified bears because they're hot . . . there is a particular way that butch fat women carry themselves that is so specific and so beautiful."

Not everyone who is attracted to fat bodies is attracted to all fat bodies. Of course, not everyone who is attracted to thin bodies is attracted to all thin bodies, either. But because being attracted to fat bodies is so taboo in our culture—not unusual, mind you, just taboo—many people jump to the conclusion that if you're attracted to one fat body you're attracted to them all or that bigger is necessarily better in your eyes. This simply isn't so. Just as there are people who are attracted to thinner bodies but still find some thin bodies too thin for their tastes, there are people who are attracted to fatter ones but only those within a certain range of fatness. Some like very fat partners, others like medium fat partners, still others prefer partners who are just over the border of plumpness, and, yes, there are some for whom bigger is categorically better. And still tastes vary. There are "leg men" and aficionados of broad shoulders and bubble butts, there are people who really love thunder thighs and big bellies and soft, pillowy expanses of breasts. There is as much variation in tastes among people who are attracted to fatter bodies as there is among people who are attracted to thinner ones.

Some, but not all, people who are attracted to fat bodies consider their attraction to be along the lines of a sexual orientation, a defining characteristic of what they like and who they are sexually. Some of these folks refer to themselves as *fat admirers*, or FAs for short. *FA* often refers primarily to straight men who like fat women, who are often referred to as *BBW*, for *big beautiful women*. Variations on the theme include *FFA*, or *female fat admirer*, for straight women who like fat men, or *BHMs* (*big handsome men*). *Chubby chaser* or just *chaser* is used in the lesbian, gay, bisexual, transgender, intersex (LGBTI) community to refer to a gay man who likes fat guys. Some fans of gay male *bears*— hairier, more traditionally masculine and beefy guys—also like their bears fat. BBW/ FA folks, chubs/chasers, and bears have all developed their own subcultures, too, complete with dedicated social clubs and

> "I love love love big, thick thighs. My earliest form of masturbation was straddling a tree branch and rocking against it; I love riding a partner's thigh in a similar way, and larger thighs feel better for that."

events, websites, porn, weekend getaway "bashes" at hotels and resorts, and more. So much for "no one is attracted to fat people"!

Myth:
Fat men have tiny penises.

Busted! Whether the man is fat or thin, tall or short, pale skinned or dark skinned, the average penis is between 5 and 7 inches long when erect. Penis size is largely the result of genetics. Fatness can't influence genetics (although genetics do influence fatness), so it's not as if someone's penis-size genes change when they gain weight. So some fat men certainly do have small penises. But some fat men have big ones. It's pretty much the luck of the draw.

What lies behind the oft-repeated myth of the fat guy with the little dick is actually a simple problem of perspective. Put a carrot on a great big serving tray, and it's going to look mighty puny. Put the same carrot on a dinner plate, and it'll look normal. Move it to a saucer, and it'll look gigantic. Fat guys are bigger, in proportion to their penises, than thin guys. A 6-inch penis is still 6 inches no matter what, but it doesn't look as big against a bigger body.

What also may be at issue, depending on the man, how fat he is, and where and how his body stores fat, is fat padding around the pubic area. The region around the pubic bone is one of the places where bodies can store fat. The upper thighs, likewise, are common fat repositories. In men who store a lot of fat in these places, fat padding can make the penis seem shorter than it is. In some cases, a change of position—for instance, lying on the back—can allow the flesh in the area a little more room to spread out, lessening the degree to which the functional length of the penis is affected by fat.

> "Fat men tend to have well-padded pubic regions that hit my clit really well during some penis-in-vagina (PIV) positions; I generally have an easier time orgasming from PIV with fat partners as a result."

Some people find that these fat deposits aren't a problem at all. Some people are actually big fans of these particular fleshy bits and find them distinctly useful!

Myth:
All fat women are easy; they're desperate.

Busted! I won't lie, it can sometimes be hard for a fat person to find a date in this fat-phobic culture, and both loneliness and the fear of being undesirable or unlovable can be hard to live with. When these things are in play, and a sexual opportunity comes along, it can seem like a really good idea to go for it, especially if it seems to be accompanied by a little bit of tenderness and kindness. Sometimes it turns out that it is a good idea to go for it. Other times you leap at a chance that ends up being a bad idea in the long run. Either way, this is hardly limited to fat people, and for better or worse, it's a very human thing to do. A long dry spell, or merely the threat of one, can bring out feelings of desperation in just about anyone.

That being said, assuming that anyone, fat or otherwise, is desperate for your attention is beyond rude and puts a person well into the realm of being an arrogant jackass. Just because you *think* someone else is the kind of person who might be desperate doesn't mean they actually are.

As for the despicable, abusive, and immature practice known as *hogging*, where men seek to take advantage (usually for one another's entertainment) of what they believe to be fat women's sexual desperation by picking up and fucking the fattest woman they can find on a given night, the less said the better. It's hateful, cruel, exploitive, and misogynist in the extreme, and it should be soundly condemned by anyone with a shred of respect for their fellow human beings.

"I think there's a certain belief among men that if they hit on the fat girl, she'll be so overcome with gratitude/desperation that she'd never think to say no to anything he wanted. When these men find out that isn't the case, they can be incredibly cruel and that quickly becomes a pretty hurtful experience. I used to really internalize that, but now I realize what a load of crap that is."

Myth:
Fat women have so many folds and rolls that you can't even find their pussies; you just have to slap a thigh and ride the wave in.

Busted! If you can see another person's head and feet and still not figure out where the genitals should be, I think a refresher course in human anatomy is in order. Plus, whenever I hear people say things like this, I always think it sounds more like they're expressing a fantasy that they're afraid of (surfing on waves of warm, soft, sexy flesh!). Paging Dr. Freud . . . your slip is showing!

Myth:
Fat people become fat because they're hiding from sex.

Busted! Fat people become fat for many reasons. Genetics, upbringing, endocrine issues, chronic illness, eating habits, movement levels, disability, medications, and much else—in addition to psychological factors—can influence weight. It's common that more than one of these factors will be in play at any given time. The reasons why any given person is fat—or thin—simply aren't always clear or easy to decipher.

Coping with stress is very much an individual thing. Some people tend to look for ways to hide from sex and other stressful things, like family drama or romantic rejection or job hunting, while other people seem wired for directness. Avoidance is a pretty normal, common behavior where scary and difficult issues are involved. Emotional eating may be entwined with avoidance, or vice versa. Or it may not. Some fat folks are emotional eaters; others are not. And, likewise, some emotional eaters are fat, while others are not.

In the end, it's none of your business why someone is fat or what their personal psychological issues may be. You don't need to know why someone is fat any more than you need to know why someone is bald or blind or left-handed or tall: a person is a person, not a puzzle you have to solve. Treat the person accordingly.

Myth:
Fat women have huge vaginas.

Busted! Sorry to burst your junior comedian bubble, but no, fat women do not rent their vaginas out as pup tents during the off season. Just like fat men don't all magically have small penises, fat women don't all magically have huge vaginas. (And, anyway, why would fat make penises small but vaginas large? It doesn't make sense!) As is the case with penises, vaginas are more similar than they are different, and their dimensions—insofar as you can talk about the dimensions of a tube whose walls are normally collapsed in against each other unless something is placed inside it—are determined by genetic lottery.

All vaginas have the built-in capacity to stretch, a necessary trait for the birthing of babies. Their muscular walls also have the built-in capacity to squeeze. (Whether fat or thin or in between, women who want to improve the muscle tone of their pelvic muscles, including those that surround the barrel of the vagina, can do Kegel exercises, which systematically squeeze and release these muscles and build their strength.) In general, however, the at-rest dimensions of vaginas, as well as their innate elasticity and muscle tone, vary somewhat from woman to woman just like the size and shape of earlobes or fingers or any other genetic trait.

Myth:
Being attracted to fat partners encourages those partners to maintain an unhealthy lifestyle, and people who get into long-term relationships with fat people are courting heartbreak because their fat partners will die young.

Busted! Let's just cut to the chase here. The above are not statements of fact; they are code. Translation: Love and health are magical rewards for doing things right. You know, like when people do the whole having-a-body thing "right" by not being fat—because, as we all know, thin people always, but always, find perfect and everlasting love, never get sick, and live forever.

Rrrrrright.

This is sizeist prejudice, plain and simple. The truth, as performance artist Glenn Marla puts it, is that there is no wrong way to have a body. People just have them, in all their vast diversity and changeability. People who have bodies sometimes fall in love or have people fall in love with them. Love is not a reward. It is a gift. The difference between a reward and a gift is that rewards must be earned, but gifts are given.

Similarly, people who have bodies also sometimes become injured, disabled, or ill. These are physical events and circumstances, not forms of punishment. Unfortunately for the people who like to think that their own personal goodness will protect them from such physical events, there is no actual moral lesson in it when someone gets cancer or kidney disease or has a heart attack or is hit by a bus: these things happen to the fat and the thin, the young and the old, the "healthy" and the "unhealthy," and for that matter to the kind and the unkind, the honorable and the despicable. Furthermore, like it or not, every last one of us, no matter how perfect a paragon of virtue we manage to be, is going to die some day. Life is an incurable, 100-percent-fatal sexually transmitted disease that you get from your parents. No one, not even skinny people, gets out alive.

Are there connections between how we behave and what happens to us, both in terms of love and in terms of health? Sure there are. Spit in the face of everyone you encounter and you will dramatically decrease the odds that one of them is going to want to ask you out on a date (although there are some people who like that sort of thing). Smoke three packs of unfiltered cigarettes every day and you will dramatically increase the odds that eventually you will suffer from lung disease, although a risk is still not a certainty.

That someone is attracted to fat people, on the other hand, can not meaningfully increase or decrease the odds that any particular other person will be, or become, fat. Our culture puts a lot of emphasis on the idea that people will try to change their bodies for the purpose of being found sexy or loveable. This is what drives the lion's share of the multibillion-dollar weight-loss industry, after all. But there is no reason to assume that people will try to become fatter just because they find out that there are some people in the world who are attracted to fat partners. Not only is there an entire culture of anti-fat prejudice that pretty effectively silences this idea, but most people, including people who are already fat, aren't actually interested in deliberately getting fatter. Back in the Victorian era, sure, women sometimes struggled to become a bit plumper, the better to fill out a bosomy corset. But that was a long time ago. The likelihood that a person is going to get fatter just because some theoretical sexual partner *might* be attracted to fat partners is, if you'll pardon the pun, vanishingly slim.

Additionally, the notion that if a fat person finds love while fat, it will remove all incentive for them to lose weight is laughably short-sighted. Being loved, or in a relationship, doesn't switch off the ability to make decisions about one's own life. Nor does it protect fat people from still having to live and interact in a fat-despising world, which provides its own "incentives" against weight gain. There is no truth to the idea that accepting fat people makes them fatter, no more than there is a shred of support for the notion that being the object of disgust and hatred makes people thinner. If disgust and hatred worked that way, there'd be far fewer fat people, wouldn't you think?

Will being loved regardless of fatness discourage people from trying to lose weight? Maybe. But maybe being loved and cherished will encourage a fat person to get regular preventive medical care and generally to want to do what they can in order to stick around longer and enjoy a good life with a loving partner, whether or not that includes any change in weight. Either way, the idea that having love or romance in one's life actively encourages bad health habits is, frankly, silly. I have never once heard anyone argue "Oh, it's bad to be attracted to smokers because it just encourages their unhealthy lifestyle," even though the link between cigarette smoking and illness is very direct and incredibly well established. It seems pretty clear that when someone spouts nonsense about how being attracted to fat people just encourages them, what they really mean is, "Oh my God, how could you possibly think of rewarding someone who is *doing it wrong?!*"

Health and longevity are complicated things, and there are many, many contributing factors—genetics, environment, pollution and toxins, stress, exercise, nutrition—to whether someone lives a long and/or healthy life. There is a lot we don't know about how it all works. One of the things we do know, though, is that loving relationships appear to promote longevity and strong social relationships can buffer the mental and physical effects of aging. If people were as truly invested in the health and well-being of others as they pretend to be, they wouldn't say that being inclined to love and be in relationships with fat people "encourages unhealthy lifestyles." Instead they'd tell the truth and say that loving and being loved is fantastic for your health and longevity, no matter what your size.

Myth:
Fat people are lazy lovers because it's too much effort for them to work at it.

Busted! Fat people aren't necessarily lazy, and as one of my ex-bosses proved every day of his lousy, scrawny life, lazy people aren't necessarily fat. Even if they were, it wouldn't necessarily matter when it comes to sex. I've known more than a few people who, if asked to walk a mile to the store or scrub a floor on their hands and knees, would react as if I'd asked them to kick a puppy. But these same people would be delighted to jump into bed with an attractive partner and shag the night away with moves that practically qualified them for Cirque du Soleil. It seems that sex can be pretty motivating. Who knew?

There's nothing wrong with being a pillow princess, just lying back and enjoying a lover's attention, as long as everyone's getting what they want out of the experience. But there's no reason to assume that a fat person, or any person, will go that route.

It also bears mentioning that the whole "fat people are lazy lovers" thing pretty much contradicts the whole "fat girls try harder because they have to" myth. They're both wrong, as it happens, but they sure as hell can't both be right.

Myth:
*If you sleep with a fat person, you'll
get crushed, smothered, or worse.
I saw it on CSI, so it must be true!*

Busted! People can be clumsy, they can misgauge their movements, and sometimes one person moves when another person thought the partner was going to stay still and the result is a clonk and a resounding Ow! Accidental sex-related injury happens to us all: I've been joking for over a decade now that I should write a sex handbook entitled *How Not to Break Your Nose on Someone Else's Pubic Bone*. In some cases, accidental collisions with fatter or heavier partners can be more injurious than they would be with thinner ones because there's more weight behind the collision. But this varies based on the physics of the individual situation and is not always true.

What people always seem to imagine will happen is that a fat woman on top of a thinner man will squash him flat. Funny how no one seems to worry about this when it's some 280-pound, six-foot-four linebacker type getting on top of a petite little 100-pound woman, though, isn't it? It's not about the weight difference between partners, in other words, or even about the size difference. It's about the idea that women are supposed to be smaller than men and about the sense that fat cannot be trusted—that it's out to get you. It's also about an unfounded fear that fat people are invariably physically weak and would be unable to hold themselves up or move themselves off of a partner if the partner were in discomfort or distress.

Relax. Fat is not out to get you. It is not even contagious. And, as fat people can demonstrate quite readily, many of us are really quite strong. Think of it this way: a thin person has to go to the gym to leg-press 300 pounds, but a fat person may only have to stand up from a chair. In a pinch, if a fat person is on top and the person on the bottom is uncomfortable, the person on top can always roll off to one side. Fat people are simply not going to overpower you with their massive chub and then have no way whatsoever to get themselves off of you. And you, Freakedout McScaredpants, are not so weak and frail that you couldn't at the very least struggle to let them know you were in distress. That's pretty much all there is to that.

Honestly, the more I hear this old canard, the more I think it sounds like another one of those fantasies masquerading as a fear: Oh no, Br'er Rabbit, please don't throw me into that briar patch! Don't immobilize me during sex! Oh, no, I'm pinned down under this sexy naked fat person and I can't get away! Whatever shall I do? Eeek! (For more on this, and advice about getting on top when you're fat, see page 175.)

Myth:
Fat people stink and are filthy, especially their crotches.

Busted! People who don't wash get stinky. People who don't clean themselves get filthy. Crotches can be particularly pungent no matter the person's size: an abundance of sweat glands, skin oil glands, and various other secretions coupled with a hothouse environment with poor ventilation can equal a galloping case of BO for even the skinniest person.

Fortunately, soap does not have a weight limit. Water is one size fits all. And even for people who may have trouble getting to those hard-to-reach spots—something that can be caused by injury, illness, or disability as well as fatness—there are tools like handheld showers, back brushes and sponges, bidets, and so on, all engineered to help people stay fresh and comfortable and clean.

Average diligence to personal hygiene is enough for most fat people, just as it is for most thinner folks. If it isn't, and you're noticing odor problems on a frequent basis when there aren't extenuating factors like hot summer weather or a massive case of nerves triggering excess sweating, consider seeing a doctor about it. See "Cleanliness Is Next to Sexiness," page 40, for more on this issue.

Myth:
Fat women love to give oral sex because obviously they're orally fixated.

Busted! Have you ever noticed that no one says this about smokers? That should tell you something. The myth that fat people are fat because they cannot seem to stop shoveling food into their mouths is just that, a myth. Sure, some people—fat and thin—adore giving head. For others, it's not quite as far up on their list of things they like to do. Some people find it off-putting. Like many other sexual things, there's a spectrum, and where one falls on that spectrum hasn't a single thing to do with what one weighs.

SURVEY SAYS:

What's your favorite thing about having sex with fat people?

"Big breasts, big hips, big asses, great curves. Don't need to worry about 'breaking' your partner during sex or rough play."

"He made me feel small and delicate. That was nice. He was a very substantial man."

"I love touching and feeling the textures and contours and hidden folds of their body. I love being with someone bigger

continued

---

than me because I feel protected. I like being with someone big because I don't worry so much that I will injure them."

"As a fat person myself, I enjoy being with someone who can match my weight; I'm less afraid of being too heavy for comfort. I've been with partners that are significantly smaller than me, and I've worried about crushing them! I also enjoy the softness and fullness of a fat partner; I find a soft body more sensual to the touch."

"I personally like the feel of fleshiness. I also like transgression and the sort of political act of implicitly declaring fat women worthwhile partners."

"The first time my partner fucked me, it was with his belly and his fat. It was AMAZING. I had never experienced fat like that before."

"The feeling! I love big, soft parts (on women). I also like the weight on top of me, although many partners feel uncomfortable doing that. Further, I've had a history of having highly orgasmic partners, and I understand that some studies show that fat women are more likely to be orgasmic. It's unclear whether that's related, or if perhaps something else is giving me such good fortune."

"Fat is soft and squishy and cuddly and feels wonderful to touch. Heavy partners are able to fuck me incredibly hard (which I love), partly just because of the physics involved. I can't toss a fat partner around with the ease I can with a thin partner. Although that's a neat experience too, it's lovely to be able to anchor against someone solid during sex. I love feeling that kind of anchoring weight on top of me, too."

chapter one

Body and Soul

Long before we have to make any decisions about who's getting on top, there are lots of other sex and relationship issues that have to be negotiated so we can work toward creating the love and sex lives we desire. This section deals with important issues around the intersection of the body and the self. Here you will learn about what you can and should expect from relationships, what good sex and relationships can and can't do for you, how to negotiate a variety of social issues that come up around sex and relationships when you have a bigger body, and the relationships between clothing and hygiene and your sexual self-esteem. Last but certainly not least, there are some thoughts on how sex and relationships can be affected by body changes, physical self-care, and movement, and why going on a diet might also mean that you lose out in your sex life.

What You Can Expect

It can be hard out there for a fatty. Fat people get crapped on, metaphorically speaking, a thousand times a day. Ads tell us that our bodies are icky and ugly. The shelves in the supermarket try to sell

20

us foul diet food full of dubious chemicals. Our families and friends may nag us—or worse—about our weight, about our size, about our appearance. Doctors lecture us about how we're going to die of The Fat, and they attribute our every sniffle to the fact that we're not svelte. There is always the fear that people will dump us, refuse to date us, humiliate us, or set us up for public mockery because of our size. We're punch lines and, sometimes, punching bags. It's really, tragically, horribly easy to internalize it all, to assume that fat is really as bad as everyone seems to be saying and that we deserve all the fat-hating crap that lands on our heads.

This is bullshit. It's all bullshit. But it is especially bullshit to think that you somehow deserve the mistreatment—or an unsatisfying or nonexistent love and sex life—because you're fat.

You are here. You are human. Because you are here and you are human, you have a right to dignity and decency no matter what you look like, no matter what you weigh, no matter who you are. You may or may not like being fat. You may or may not agree with mainstream views about fatness. I don't know and I don't care, and it doesn't matter. You are still here, you are still human, and you still have a right to be treated with a certain baseline of respect. That's why they call it human decency.

Unfortunately, not everyone will show you the dignity and decency you, like everyone else, deserve. As fabulous and giving and kind and loving and wonderful as human beings can be, we can also be selfish, nasty, brutal pack animals whose more civilized impulses get overridden by an ancient, survival-oriented propensity for power games. These power games, unfortunately and unkindly, mean that many people feel that gunning for fat people is a safe bet. More unfortunately, they are often correct.

Protecting yourself, by which I mean creating and enforcing boundaries that protect your mental, emotional, physical, and sexual safety, is your responsibility. This is especially important when it comes to intimate relationships, because where we are intimate, we are vulnerable. It would be your responsibility if you were thin. It is even more your responsibility if you are fat. And yes, alas, intersections of fatness and other minority statuses will mean that, if you are both fat and a member of another minority, you may have to be even more demanding, and work even harder, to get the dignity you deserve.

Neither I nor anyone else can decide where your own personal boundaries should be or how much protection you need to provide for yourself. Only you know what levels of risk are acceptable to you, how bad of a possible burn you are able to tolerate. Your tolerance of risk can and probably will change as other circumstances in your life change. You will have to periodically revisit your boundaries and make adjustments. So I cannot tell you what your boundaries should be, but here are some general guidelines specifically in relation to love and sex that can help you decide where your personal boundaries with regard to relationships and sexuality might most usefully lie.

1. *You do not have to accept bad treatment in order to get love, attention, or sex.* It is not better to be abused or mistreated than it is to be lonely. It is possible to be comfortable and happy and be solitary or celibate, and many people are. It's certainly better to fly solo than to be abused. More to the point, there are people out there who will treat you kindly and well. It may take you some time to find those people, and there may be bumps in the road along the way—this happens to everybody, of all sizes—but it is much better to take the time to seek them out than it is to settle for people who are hurtful and damaging.

2. *You do not have to put yourself at physical risk to get love, attention, or sex.* If someone you are intimate with wants you to agree to something that is physically risky for you, you don't have to do it just because they ask. This is true if a partner refuses to use contraception or refuses to use safer sex techniques, it is true if a partner wants you to do something that seems likely to result in an injury, and it is true if a partner

asks you to do something that seems like it might have bad physical consequences down the line.

This is especially important to remember in regard to things that may not seem so serious at the time, like unprotected sex. Unwanted pregnancies can happen whether you are fat or thin. The HIV virus does not care what you weigh and neither do the microorganisms that cause syphilis, gonorrhea, chlamydia, herpes, or genital warts/HPV. Anyone who refuses to be responsible in regard to these issues is not only putting themselves at risk but also putting you at risk, and chances are good that if they're putting themselves at risk with you, they've been doing the same with other people, and that's not a good thing.

Love or sex that comes with unwanted and unacceptable risks is not better than not getting love or sex at all. It's really not worth it. There is plenty of good love and positive sex out there to be had. It's worth seeking out. And it's worth not settling for less.

3. *You do not have to agree to anything that hurts you emotionally.* The desire to please a partner is understandable. So is the fear that a partner might leave if you if she doesn't get what she wants. But you do not have to let anyone do anything to you or with you that makes you sad or anxious, depressed or self-loathing, and no partner who claims to care for you should insist that you do. You may be fat, but that doesn't mean that you exist to serve other people's desires at the expense of your own equilibrium and happiness.

4. *Anyone who uses love or the promise of love to manipulate you into doing something that hurts you is abusing you and violating your trust.* Period. Any sentence that includes "if you really loved me, you'd . . ." or "prove you love me by doing . . ." has only one answer: real love does not include emotional blackmail.

5. *If your gut tells you that something is wrong or that someone is untrustworthy, it's really okay to listen to your gut.* Sometimes we subconsciously pick up on important things that don't register with our conscious minds. Sometimes we know things that we don't really want to admit to ourselves. Sometimes it's hard to trust the little inner "Spidey Sense" tingles we get from time to time. It may seem like we're reading too much into something. We might be afraid of seeming too timid, paranoid, or untrusting. We may think "it couldn't possibly be that way," even when part of us is pretty sure that it is.

   More often than not, our gut is smart and if we pay attention to it, it will save us a lot of trouble. Better safe than sorry. And if you end up feeling like a doofus because you were more cautious than you needed to be, consider that you now have more data that will help you make a better judgment call next time.

6. *You are allowed to have high standards.* Being fat does not mean you have to settle for anyone who will have you. What you want is just as important as what anyone else wants. Of course, having standards that include a little bit of wiggle room is always a good idea, because, frankly, there is a difference between high standards and standards that are so idealistic that no one can possibly measure up.

   I like to think of standards as being like the signs at amusement parks that say "You must be at least this tall to ride this ride." It's always okay to be *taller*. You are under no obligation to be a one-size-fits-all sort of person, especially when it comes to relationships. Just as with clothes, a good fit makes all the difference.

7. *You are allowed to want what you want.* Oh, it can be so hard to let yourself want things! Especially when you're fat, it can be easy to feel like you shouldn't have too much in the way of desires—that your body is already "too much" as it is. Or

people may feel that only thin people deserve to have desires or have their desires taken seriously, that this is a privilege reserved for "good" bodies. Nonsense! Whether what you want is a three-hour backrub, to have someone go down on you until you scream with ecstasy, or just a nice lunch date—or anything else, singly or in combination—your desires are every bit as valid and as worthwhile as anyone else's. Besides, they're yours, and that makes them especially valid and worthwhile for your own pleasure, fulfillment, and happiness. Of course there are no guarantees that you, or anyone, will get everything you want But as poet Robert Browning put it, "a man's reach should exceed his grasp, or what's a Heaven for?" Letting yourself want what you want, openly and honestly, gets you at least halfway to telling other people what you want. Given how few people are telepathic, that's a huge plus all by itself.

Things Would Be So Different If They Were Not as They Are

If there's one thing people are good at, it's limiting themselves for no good reason. We all do it, and we all know other people who do it: the friend who complains of overwork but refuses to consider a vacation, the friend who wants to learn to scuba dive but has dismissed it as being unaffordable without even looking into how much it would cost. But self-limitation doesn't even have to involve concrete things like a vacation or scuba diving. We do it to ourselves just as much when we indulge in thinking thoughts like "If only I were a size smaller, I'd get hit on at parties" or "If I had a lover, then I'd be able to feel more confident about my sexiness" or a million other similar things.

Fat people are particularly prone to this because of the myth we get sold daily in this culture, that fat people can't do this, they shouldn't do that, and they won't be able to do the other thing until they lose weight. We're all deeply and continually exposed to the message that life will be better, and that people will approve of our existence, when our bodies are thinner. As a result, we often don't let ourselves do things we want to do—wear a sleeveless top, travel, ask someone out on a date, and so on. We're afraid of what might happen, and we've become convinced that if we do these things as fat people, it can't possibly end well. We let the lives we want be contingent on something else. There's always something we have to achieve before we can have what we want. In this way we put what we really desire on hold.

There's just one problem with putting your life on hold: it means you're putting your life on hold. Sure, as the legendary (and often fat) comedienne Anna Russell used to sing, "Things would be so different if they were not as they are." But the truth of the matter is that at any given moment all you actually have to work with is things as they are. The only starting place you have is where you are right now.

If you're reading this book, chances are good that you are looking for some advice that will help you have a better life. Specifically, you're looking for some advice on your sex life, and your love life, and you're hoping that this book will provide encouragement and insight in those arenas. As the author, I sincerely hope I am able to provide this to you. But the single biggest thing you can do for the quality of your life, and for your happiness in every aspect of your life—including your love life and your sex life—is something only you can do, and you have to do it for yourself.

Here it is: stop putting your life on hold.

This is the central message of size acceptance philosophy and the central message of this book. Accepting that you're fat doesn't mean giving up or giving in; it just means accepting that this is the body you've got. You're fat, and that's not the end of the world. Life goes on. As you may have already noticed, it's not as if your life has actually stopped happening just because you're fat. So you might as well live it the way you want to. Wear that sexy outfit. Try that enticing sex toy. Ask that hot person out on a date. Try getting on top. Go out with your friends to that dance club. Tell your partner about your fantasy. Put up that online personal ad. Whatever it is that you've been wanting to do, give it a whirl. Why wait?

Sure, it may not be a perfect experience. Life's like that. You may end up disappointed or hurt. Those are the breaks sometimes. But not risking failure means you aren't risking success. Not taking any risks feels safe, yes, but that's only because you know exactly what the outcome will be: nothing.

I know it's terrifically easy, and terrifically tempting, to think about taking a risk and end up just taking a nap. I know it's scary to take risks, and believe me when I say that I totally know about the nightmarish jungle of what-ifs that spring up the instant you even think about doing something that's risky and frightening. But the truth is that the odds of your life magically turning into an all-singing, all-dancing road show of exactly what you want, forever and ever amen, without your having to do anything at all, are pretty damn nonexistent. On the other hand, if you do make some changes, take some risks, and see what happens, you've opened the door to possibility.

This brings me to the other huge thing that will make your love and sex life immeasurably better and will do wonders for your life in general. Again, it's something that only you can do: don't expect love and sex to heal your entire life.

Love is a many-splendored thing. Sex has the potential to be a lifelong source of joy and amazement and insight and goodness. I'd be the last person to say otherwise. There are a thousand excellent reasons to devote some time and energy to improving your love life and your sex life. But neither love nor sex is a magic pill that instantly erases every source of trouble, stress, and frustration. Love and sex certainly don't erase the various problems that go along with being fat. You can be madly in love with the perfect person and still have a hard time finding clothes that fit. You can have deliriously fantastic sex seven nights a week with a variety of delicious and charming individuals and still have random assholes shout fatphobic nastiness at you on the street. Having lots of lovely orgasms, unfortunately, cannot keep your doctor from nagging you about your weight, even if they can help you cope with how stressful it is to be nagged. Neither love nor sex will give you a reprieve from the rest of life. It only feels like it ought to, in that first heady flush of hormones and limerence. But it doesn't—not for you, not for anyone, no matter how thin or fat. Good love and sexual relationships can help you deal with the stresses of life, but they can't simply erase them.

It's easy to think that everything would be different if only you had a lover or better sex or more orgasms or someone who brought you breakfast in bed every morning. But once more we are back in the land of Things Would Be So Different If They Were Not as They Are. If you had a lover, you would have a lover. And that might very well be really wonderful. But it would not change the fact that your boss is incompetent or your sister-in-law is a high-maintenance drama queen.

If you take nothing else away from this book, take these two things: don't put your life on hold and don't expect love and sex to heal your life. Giving your fears a little less time in the driver's seat makes you more open to the possibility of good things happening in your life. Letting your experiences out of the confining cage of unrealistic expectations means you are open to lovely surprises. Not undermining the goodness of the good things in your life by trying to force them to be something they can't be means you are more likely to appreciate them for what they are. It's a good recipe for a good life. Everyone, no matter who they are or what they weigh, deserves more of that.

Physical "Fit-ness"

Fat people weigh more and take up more space than thin people. This isn't something to be ashamed of, and it isn't necessarily anything to gloat about either; it's just the way it is. It does, however, mean that when we fat folks are moving around in a world where most physical objects are designed for thinner bodies, we have to strategize about the physical aspects of where we want to go and what we want to do. This comes up not just in everyday routine but also in our love and sex lives.

Space is one concern. Chairs with arms, narrow restaurant booths, and movie theater seats seemingly designed for malnourished twelve-year-olds are common problems that might come up in the context of a date or an evening out—but so might being stuck in a car that you don't fit into comfortably or whose seat belts aren't sufficient to protect a bigger person. Although people are remarkably ingenious about making the best of the space available to them, being cramped and confined is unpleasant at best and can be embarrassing, humiliating, and physically painful at worst. I always figure that if I'm going to have bruises on my hips, I want the process of getting them to be enjoyable, not an experience I remember with grinding resentment.

Thinking ahead about what physical accommodations you might need, and asking the questions that need to be asked to make sure you'll have enough space for comfort, is important. This may seem embarrassing at first, particularly with regard to public spaces or other people's houses, though most people find it is less so over time. It might help to remember that retail and service/hospitality businesses get many special requests in the course of the average day, and yours is nowhere near the oddest one they will have gotten. In many cases, you can email instead, if you prefer, which may lessen any embarrassment you might feel. Or perhaps a date or partner can ask on your behalf, a gracious and caring gesture.

Structural stability in furnishings and the like is another concern, and one that's harder to address. Not all fat people are built the same, and therefore not every fat person will have the same worries or the same reasons to worry. It's not always possible to tell whether a fat person is big or heavy enough, or shaped in ways that might cause problems with furnishings, just by looking at them. This includes being able to tell this about yourself: our image of our own bodies is often not 100 percent accurate. (I continually think my butt is bigger than it is and am consistently surprised when a chair or turnstile or what-have-you is actually no problem at all.)

Unfortunately, not all furniture or other structures are built the same either. You may call ahead to find out whether a restaurant has armless chairs, and they may say yes, but they don't necessarily have *sturdy* armless chairs. You just can't know whether a chair or other piece of furniture will wobble, bend, or break. Folding chairs, although armless, can be treacherously flimsy, and injection-molded plastic chairs of the type so often put out at sidewalk cafes are infamously even worse. It's not funny or fun to have a chair break under you (and, yes, the plastic ones can break—there is a somewhat infamous moment in an episode of the TV program *Bizarre Foods* in which the only slightly rotund host, Andrew Zimmern, has one go to pieces beneath him on camera). Besides, it's dangerous.

Sometimes the only thing you can do is to gingerly take a test sit and see if it feels stable enough, and, if not, see what can be done to find an alternative. The same is true of things like bed frames. These are even harder to guess about, although as a general rule, the lighter the components, the more likely it is to be flimsy. I am far from the only person I know who has managed to break slats in cheap futon frames during sex. (I once managed to break one while masturbating, and it wasn't even my bed. True story. I think that there should be a merit badge for that.) It's a little surprising and a little embarrassing, yes, but not the end of the world.

If you are fat or you have sex with people who are, it is not a bad idea to take some special care to make sure that anyplace you are likely to engage in sex is both large enough and sturdy enough to handle what you're dishing out. Beds should be on sturdy frames or simply on the floor. Chairs and benches should be well built and regularly checked to make sure their joints are all solid and nothing is wiggling or wobbling. More exotic equipment, like slings and bondage furniture, should be sturdily built with attachment points that can handle considerably more stress than you think might ever be put on them. (This is actually a good idea no matter what the size of the people you play with: torque can be a harsh mistress.) This is easy to do, but it does require attention to details like sturdy grommets, materials of appropriate tensile strength (rope, fabric), and adequate structural strength in mounting surfaces, beams, walls, and so on.

If you choose to use household furnishings for sex play—bending someone over the arm of the couch, for instance—make sure that the arm of the couch is up to the task, and bear in mind that with all that weight there will not only be downward force but also a great deal of force being applied sideways, diagonally, and in other directions. Check joints and joins in furniture frames, if possible. At the very least, give things a good shove and see if there is any play in the frame. If there is, a frame may need to be tightened, reglued, or reinforced with mending plates (ask at your hardware store) before it will be genuinely safe to have sex on top of it. Some people also have good luck using rope to lash and reinforce furniture framing. If something goes to pieces after all that, you can definitely chalk it up to just being so wild and uninhibited that even the furniture couldn't handle you!

There are some fat admirers who eroticize people getting stuck in chairs or tight spaces and others who fetishize people breaking furniture because of their weight or size. "Stuck" and breakage fetishes and fantasies are not unheard of among people who like thinner bodies, either. As with most fetish interests, there are ways to play with the problems of size, fit, and sturdiness for erotic pleasure without putting anyone in any real danger of humiliation or injury. As a gift for a friend-with-benefits, a friend once had photos taken of her substantial, skimpily dressed self pressed up against the glass of an old-fashioned phone booth, as if she were trapped inside and couldn't get out. She could get out just fine, of course, but the illusion of stuckness was enthusiastically received. Such things are not, however, something that should be done without full informed consent. It is of course impolite and awkward if one person dwells fetishistically on embarrassing or unhappy experiences that another has experienced. Discretion, tact, and careful, good-humored communication are, as is the case with so much else in life, key to a pleasant experience.

There are other size and fit issues that affect sex lives. Fatter folks also have to go out of their way to find sexual accessories that are accommodating: dildo harnesses, particularly, can be tricky to find in larger sizes, but certainly not impossible (see Resource Guide for recommendations). Size, fit, and reach issues may also affect sexual positions and sex toy use. These are all discussed in their subject-specific sections.

The Shape of Things

Bodies don't just come in big or small, fat or skinny; they come in a variety of different shapes. There are people with wide shoulders and stooped shoulders, big hands and dainty ones, narrow feet and feet that are practically square, like Fred Flintstone's. Mostly, it's a matter of genetics. You can stand up as straight as a palace guard and still have sloping shoulders, and you can shove your big ol' gunboats into shoes two sizes too small and, at the end of the day, all you'll have to show for it is blisters. Some things about your body you just can't do much about. The way people's bodies carry fat is definitely one of those things.

There seems to be some myth, lurking in the backs of many people's minds that when people get fat, it sort of settles on their bodies evenly, all over, like a soft, sifted blanket of snow. In reality, bodies don't accumulate fat evenly all over like that. They accumulate fat in particular places, and as with foot size and shoulder curve and so on, how fat accumulates on any given body seems to be mostly a matter of genetics. The degree to which we are likely to notice someone's fat-distribution patterns often depends on how much fat there is. The fatter the body, the more exaggerated and obvious the fat patterns can become.

How much fat gets deposited where is not something that people can control. You can do all the sit-ups in the world, and if you are genetically predisposed to carry weight in your midsection, then that's exactly where you're going to carry it if you've got any to carry. It does not matter how strong or toned the underlying layer of muscles might be. A woman who normally carries her weight in her hips and thighs is not going to wake up one morning to discover that she has suddenly become a woman who carries most of her weight in her belly. You might be able to fight City Hall, but you can't fight your genes.

The places that we carry our fat, how the fat shapes itself, and how much fat accumulates in different places on the body are not things over which we have much control. This makes it all the more curious, and not a little bit problematic, that we tend to read so much into different body shapes. Some body shapes, and some patterns of fat distribution, are considered more attractive than others. They tend to be interpreted as suggesting particular things about gender and even about sexual orientation. Fairly or unfairly, reasonably or unreasonably, a lot can ride on what is nothing more than a combination of fat plus genetics.

Fat bodies are often described as existing in three basic versions. These three basic body shapes are considered by many to represent a fairly stringent hierarchy of attractiveness and gender.

Hourglass: This exaggerated version of the classic female silhouette is big in the bust, smaller in the waist, and big again in the hips and/or butt. Hourglass-shaped women are often seen as being more feminine or more womanly than women with non-hourglass shapes. Sometimes hourglass-shaped women are presumed to be heterosexual even when they aren't, because of the exaggerated femininity of their figures.

Because it is a version of the "ideal" feminine figure, the hourglass shape can bring a certain amount of privilege along with it. Hourglass-shaped women may find that their body shape allows them to be socially accepted more easily than fat women with bodies of other shapes, even if they are of similar actual weights. Our culture highly values big breasts and curvy hips in women.

"I have a pronounced hourglass shape and I sometimes wish I didn't. I get attention I don't want and I have a hard time knowing what to do with it. It still doesn't really make sense to me that this happens, as I am quite fat. I suppose fat in the "right" places makes all the difference."

Having an hourglass shape is great if you're inclined toward the kind of feminine gender presentation that our culture associates with Coke-bottle curves. It can be miserable, however, if you are not. Some women find their hourglass shapes to be nothing but trouble, because of the ways that onlookers make assumptions about their gender, their preferences, and their attitudes on the basis of the shape of their bodies. Butch women and transmasculine people with biologically female bodies can have particular problems coping with an hourglass shape.

Pear: The bottom-heavy silhouette, in which most of a person's fat is carried in the hips, butt, thighs, and lower abdomen, is known as the "pear shape." It can be seen as feminine, although not as feminine as the hourglass. Men who are pear shaped often find that the "hippy" qualities of this body shape mean that they are perceived as not fully masculine, as they suggest a feminine broadness in the hips. Sometimes observers may—correctly or incorrectly—assume that a man who is pear shaped is gay, because he has a "feminine" body shape. A pear shape can be an asset to transfeminine people, since it enhances the ability to suggest feminine curves. Sexually speaking, the pear shape is sometimes fetishized, just like the hourglass can be. People who are particularly fond of big butts and heavy thighs can be intensely attracted to pear-shaped bodies.

"Being a bottom heavy man sucks! It's like the anti-chick magnet. I had one woman tell me she figured I was gay because I had hips. I thought 'Of course I have hips, doesn't everybody?'"

In some cases, the pear shape can be a sign of a medical problem. Lipedema is a medical condition in which fat deposits in a distinctive pattern, from waist to ankles, in the lower half of the body, and creates major problems for lymphatic drainage, leading to pain and vastly increased potential for infections and other issues. It is found almost exclusively in women and is often misdiagnosed. Lipedema is covered in more detail in chapter 5, To Your Health!, on page 155.

Apple: The apple body shape is one where most fat is carried in the torso, and particularly in the belly. It is the classic male pattern for fat deposition, although a fair proportion of women are also apple shaped. Because it is associated with male body shapes, it is masculinizing. We give the apple-shaped male belly all kinds of masculine nicknames—"beer belly," "biker belly," "Buddha belly"—and often talk about it with a certain bravado as a symbol of the good life. There are, for instance, a number of delis across the United States called "The Big Belly Deli." For those attracted to fat men, the belly is often a visually enticing source of erotic pleasure.

Apple-shaped women have a more difficult time. Because the apple shape is interpreted as masculine, apple-shaped women may feel as if they are less feminine, or other people may treat them as if they are. Apple-shaped women have sometimes been assumed to be lesbians, even if they aren't, because their bodies seem masculine.

In general, there are fewer people who value apple-shaped women sexually than there are people who value apple-shaped men. Apple-shaped women may feel like they are sexually invisible because of this. On the other hand, an apple shape can be an asset to butch women and transmasculine people.

As with the pear shape, there are cases in which the apple shape is a sign of an underlying medical issue. In women, being apple shaped can be part of an endocrine and metabolic condition called poly-cystic ovary syndrome (PCOS). PCOS is covered in more detail in chapter 5, To Your Health!, on page 153. The apple shape has been statistically correlated with a higher degree of cardiovascular problems; however, it is not entirely clear what the nature of that relationship is or what that might mean for health care.

> "I sort of feel that as a black woman it's more 'okay' to have an hourglass-shaped body as opposed to a stick thin body. But the idea that it's 'okay' for black women to have apple-shaped bodies is not true."

Dressing the Part

Except for the fact that you usually take them off somewhere along the way, it might seem like clothes don't have a lot to do with sex. But clothes have enormous impact on how we feel about ourselves and what kinds of impressions we make on people as we move through the world. We use them to attract, to distract, and definitely to adver-tise. Clothes are part of how we attract attention and part of how we keep it, part of how we tell the world what kind of person we are and what kind of person we're likely to be interested in. We use them to show off and seduce as well as to fool the eye and conceal. When you feel like you're not well dressed, you're likely to be less confident and might even feel embarrassed to be seen in public. When you're wearing something that makes you feel pulled together and sexy, on the other hand, you feel good and it shows.

This isn't always easy to do, though. Plus-size fashion has come a long way from the polyester double-knit ghettoes of yesteryear but, even now, the options available—particularly for those at the higher end of the weight spectrum—can leave quite a bit to be desired. Even assuming you've found clothes that have all the right stuff, it can be scary to wear things that call attention to yourself and to the way you look. Blogger and author Lesley Kinzel is a dedicated clotheshorse. She would love to see more fat people taking fashion and using it more powerfully, but she notes that it's not necessarily simple: "Willfully drawing attention to yourself with risky choices can be so terrifying, especially if you've spent much of your life invested in the idea that your body should be invisible, hidden, a source of shame. But taking risks is the only way we can learn anything new about ourselves—in this case, how we can handle putting our bodies out there in a flagrant violation of cultural expectations." She recommends taking it slowly, trying small changes, and building your comfort level one individual challenge at a time.

A great exercise that uses clothes to help you get more comfortable with and in your body is Kinzel's "white tank top" exercise. It consists of putting on a white tank top and wearing it for ten minutes every day in front of a full-length mirror. "Take in your shape, your arms, legs, face. Look for the things you like, and learn to like the things you don't, until you learn to see your own beauty first, before you see any so-called imperfections." It is, as Kinzel reminds us, our "imperfections" that make us interesting—and beautiful. "If you can feel sexy in a white tank top," she adds, "then you can feel sexy in anything."

One of the biggest problems we fat folks have with sexy clothes isn't what to wear, but where to get it. You can be sexy and pulled together and look fantastic in almost anything, but finding specifically sexy clothes, lingerie, and the like can be very difficult indeed, particularly if you wear larger than a 3X. The Resource Guide has

continued on page 40

INTERVIEW:
Playing Dress-Up with Lesley Kinzel

Lesley Kinzel was one of the fat founding mothers behind the community and blog Fatshionista. She analyzes popular culture, writes things (her book on fat issues is due out from the Feminist Press at CUNY in 2012), wears dresses, and blogs about social justice and fattery at TwoWholeCakes.com.

Q: *If you had to distill your philosophy of "fatshion" down to just a sentence or two, what would it be?*

A: Fatshion for me is about refusing to be invisible. I dress expressly to draw attention, thereby to make a statement that I am not to be ignored or dismissed. Sometimes, in a more aggressive vein: that I am fully capable of fucking you up, that my purpose is to fuck you up, even just mentally, by crashing through your expectation of how a fat person is supposed to present hirself* to the world.

Q: *What advice would you give to a fat person who was trying to dress to impress someone romantically/sexually?*

A: You will, invariably, look hottest in whatever you FEEL hottest in. If garter belts and cutout bras don't do it for you, it's going to show. And who the hell wrote the law that said only those items are sexy? If you feel most sexified in a white a-shirt and boxers, or in an oversize T-shirt, or in nothing at all, then your confidence and—probably more importantly—your comfort in your body will shine through. Few things make a person more attractive than being able to witness their comfort in their own skin.

....

*"Hir, " "sie," and "hirself" are gender-neutral pronouns that are becoming increasingly popular. "Hir" replaces "him or her," "sie" replaces "he or she," and "hirself" replaces "him- or herself."

Q: *What are some clothes strategies for the apple-shaped girl? It seems like all the sexy and trendy stuff is cut for bodies that are not apple shaped.*

A: Indeed. Actually I'd take that a step further and say our very concepts of "sexy" and "trendy" are in opposition to the apple shaped. When in recent memory has a prominent belly been in vogue? Have we ever elevated a feminine beauty standard that didn't include a distinct waist? My advice for apples is to fuck the system and wear what you like. I am partial to dresses with voluminous skirts, but there are some fatshionista bloggers out there who are traditional apples and who also work out the sheath dresses and pencil skirts like nobody's business. Clothing should showcase your body and your style—if you feel good in it, then wear it. Never be afraid to try something on, and never assume a particular style cannot work for you.

Q: *How much do you think people really notice clothes and fashion choices? Does it genuinely make a difference to your romantic/sexual prospects?*

A: My partner says today that part of why he first noticed me was because of my style—I was a fat girl wearing low-cut tops, mini-skirts, and Dr. Martens boots as a daily uniform at the time. I think fashion can be a means of drawing initial attention for some people, but ultimately attraction happens on a deeper level. Our style, how we present ourselves to the world, does say something about us, and certainly that can draw folks who like what they see. But you don't have to wear "sexy" clothing to look like someone worth talking to: I was hit on far more often while wearing totally nonsexy T-shirts for obscure bands than when I was all fishnetted and bustier-ed up for the club.

some suggestions for vendors that sell sexy clothing and have come recommended by survey and by word of mouth. Online clearing-houses like Etsy.com and eBay.com are also good resources where truly unusual items sometimes pop up. Another possibility is to have things custom made. This need not be prohibitively expensive; Etsy .com is a great place to hunt for a craftsperson who will happily work with you to create exactly what you want to wear at prices that may be less than you imagined.

Whatever you feel sexiest in will, without question, be the sexiest thing you can wear. It really doesn't matter what it is. If you feel sexiest in the nude, then by all means show off that birthday suit (as long as it won't get you arrested)! If what makes you feel like a million bucks is a pristine white T-shirt, a pair of blue jeans, and a freshly shined pair of boots, then your body language and pleasure in your own looks will convey that to the people who see you. Sleek black tights and an acid-green minidress? A glitzy Western suit worthy of the Country Music Awards? Head-to-toe black leather? A lightly starched dress shirt, really good cuff links, and a Harris tweed jacket? Whatever makes you feel like an unstoppable sex machine is fair game for "sexy clothes," because what you feel, you will reflect.

Cleanliness Is Next to Sexiness

We've all heard the old wives' tale that fat people are dirty, that we smell, that our various folds and crevices are rank and dank and unkempt and nasty. Some people even seem to think—although it makes no sense at all—that it is in fact physically impossible for fat people to be properly clean. The implication, of course, is that sex with fat people is disgusting because fat people are smelly and dirty.

Well, the truth of the matter is that from time to time, all of us are smelly and dirty. Personal cleanliness is, even for the skinniest and most scrupulous, an ongoing matter requiring regular maintenance. There are times when, no matter how lithe one is, one is bound to become sweaty and smelly and generally unappetizing. I have been with more than one thin person whose crotches were, shall we say, more fragrant than one might ideally prefer. Getting dirty and smelly is a human thing, not a fat thing.

The solution, fortunately, is simple. Wash! Wash early, wash often. If sexy naked times are on the immediate horizon, wash with a friend! Plain, mild soap and water will take care of most typical body odors, sweat, and general everyday ookiness. Dry well with a clean towel afterward, and off you go!

Although you should feel free to douse yourself in deodorants and antiperspirants and powder and lotion and perfume and aftershave if that's what you like when you're heading out or going to work or whatever, you'll want to avoid these if you are washing in order to be clean for sex. These cosmetics often taste foul, and most are not actually recommended for ingestion anyhow. Going to nibble someone's neck and getting a mouthful of Chanel No. 5, as I discovered in a most inconvenient way, is not a pleasant surprise. It may smell great, but it tastes awful. Don't be worried about smelling like your own sweet self. Bodies are not supposed to be completely tasteless and odorless. We are human beings, and our bodies are supposed to smell and taste like clean, healthy, happy bodies. This is normal and okay and, indeed, sexy: scientists have shown that people's sexual responses are affected strongly by the smells of their partners' bodies.

Some people may have trouble reaching all the parts of their bodies. Sometimes this is due to fatness, but (and I speak from personal experience), having a bad case of tennis elbow can make a proper scrub down difficult too. Arthritis, joint problems, shoulder surgery, and other ailments can also make it really difficult to reach everything you want to reach. Whatever the reason, there are workarounds that can make bath time easier and better.

First and foremost is the handheld shower. There are versions that can be connected permanently to typical wall shower fixtures, as well as versions that attach to bath taps on a temporary basis. It's convenient to be able to direct the water exactly where you want it, and especially nice to make sure you can thoroughly rinse all the nooks and crannies of the bigger body. Back brushes allow for a long, leisurely reach for scrubbing whatever parts of you might enjoy a nice brisk washing, and they help to exfoliate as well, as do the 3-foot-long Salux wash-cloths from Japan that are available at many Asian grocery stores. On a similar but gentler theme, you can find back-brush-type tools that have sponge pads instead of bristles and even ones with lotion applicators. (See Resource Guide for some places to find these.)

The genitals and anus, of course, are particularly relevant to sex. They can also be particularly tricky to keep clean if you have reach issues. Just like there are back brushes and long-handled sponges, there are also specially made long-handled tools to help you wipe after using the toilet. These can be used with toilet paper, or with pre-moistened wipes intended for toilet use.

Bidets, although uncommon in North America, are everyday fixtures in much of the rest of the world, and they are brilliant for the quick and easy cleaning of the whole genital-anal area. Bidets are normally used in addition to wiping with toilet paper, not as a substitute, but for people whose reach problems prevent them from wiping with toilet paper, a bidet can, if used diligently, get the job done. If adding a separate bidet to your bathroom is not in the cards, you might consider an attachment that turns your existing toilet into a toilet-bidet. There are companies making automated bidet attachments for standard toilets, and there are even low-tech portable hand-pump versions available. Of course, bidets are superb for post-sex washing-up as well, not just the pre-game. People of all sizes, all around the world, use bidets happily every single day.

Dealing with skin folds and creases is a special cleanliness concern that thin people just don't have to worry about as much. Because skin folds, deep navels, and deep creases in areas like the groin trap sweat and sloughed-off skin cells, and because the air circulation is limited or nonexistent, they can get particularly smelly and unpleasant in warm weather or after exercise. These moist, warm zones are ideal breeding grounds for skin infections, especially fungal ones. Such infections are not, of course, limited to fat people, as the sheer number of athlete's foot and jock itch products on the market ought to tell you. Still, the folds and creases of a fatter body do create a built-in risk for these infections, and monitoring them for signs of unwelcome life on a routine basis is a very good idea.

The skin inside skin folds and creases is soft and delicate. It is more prone to irritation than tougher skin on other parts of your body, like your hands or arms. Because the skin is so tender, it can be easy for infections to take hold, and also for scratching, rubbing, or overly vigorous scrubbing to create abrasions and scrapes that can, in turn, get infected also.

When you are washing, you should take the time to wash every inch of yourself, including the insides of skin folds and creases. It's good to keep tabs with your hands on what's going on with your entire body, including the bits you might not actually be able to see very well, so that you notice when something suspicious shows up, like a lump, bump, or sore that might need medical attention. (Pro tip: The shower is also a fantastic place for a breast self-exam or a testicle self-exam, since wet, slippery skin makes it easier and more comfortable.)

You'll want to dry off just as thoroughly when you're done. A hairdryer with a "no heat" setting is a fabulous way to thoroughly dry skin folds and creases, but don't give in to temptation and jack up the heat on the theory that it'll get you drier faster. It will, but it's also drying and potentially damaging to the already delicate skin inside those creases, and it is possible to burn yourself, as I know from particularly ouchy experience.

If you notice a persistent smell coming from any particular bit of your skin, whether a fold, crease, or otherwise, it may indicate a skin infection. Sometimes they itch, sometimes they don't; sometimes there is discharge, sometimes there isn't. There are different kinds of microorganisms that can cause skin infections, but fungal infections are most common. Mild fungal infections can often be treated at home by carefully washing and drying the affected skin, and doing your best to keep it dry, since without moisture, the fungi can't grow. Cornstarch or baby powder helps absorb moisture. Some people also have good luck with herbal remedies featuring plants known for their antifungal or antimicrobial effects. Tea tree oil is especially popular but should be diluted with some other neutral oil (almond or jojoba), because it can be harsh. Goldenseal and Oregon Grape root are other good, highly effective, antimicrobial agents with which I and others have had great success for topical use. Do make a point to talk to a trained herbalist about these options if you can, since herbs are chemical agents too, and some can be irritating or dangerous if not used properly. You can also try over-the-counter remedies for jock itch, which usually contain a low concentration of antimicrobial drugs, sufficient to get rid of low-grade infections of certain (mostly fungal) types.

If these solutions don't work, or if you just don't want to mess around with them, go to your health care provider, who can more accurately identify the infection and give you prescription drugs that can knock out the infection. Keeping things clean and dry will help discourage a repeat infection as well as keeping you sweet smelling and sweet tasting for any paramours who might happen by.

When Your Body Changes

You don't have to change your body to have fantastic, mind-blowing sex. You don't have to change your body to find love. You certainly don't have to change your body to have a vibrant and happy sensual and emotional existence. Being confident and happy in your own skin is possible, and wonderful, no matter what size you are.

But—and this can be a pretty significant *but*—bodies change whether we want them to or not. Weight can go up and down for many reasons, including sickness, depression, metabolic malfunction, and eating disorders, not just from dieting or exercising. Likewise, muscle can be gained or lost for many reasons. The size of individual body areas may shift around somewhat from time to time even if there's no change in weight. Illness, injury, surgery, medications, pregnancy and childbirth, accidents, and aging are among the many things that can cause noticeable body change.

You can be comfortable in your body at any point, in any configuration, at any size. And you can feel sexual and vital and delicious and delightful at any size or shape or ability (or disability) level, too. But feeling good and sexy about yourself at one bodily status doesn't mean you're going to be instantly comfortable if that changes.

When your body gets bigger or smaller or just changes shape, it can take your self-image and your emotional sense of self a while to catch up. Losing that sense of the familiar, and feeling like you can't depend on your body to stay the same, can be confusing and alienating. Complicated emotional reactions are common: you might feel pleased at becoming more muscular, for instance, and at the same time feel weirdly conspicuous or worry about what other people think of the change. Even changes that you look forward to or maybe even work toward intentionally—maybe you've been wanting bigger biceps for years and have been working out to get them— can feel weird sometimes.

"I'm dealing with a weird thing wherein because I was a dancer, and lithe and flexible (about 50–70 pounds ago), I sometimes think I cannot possibly still be attractive to people who knew me then. The reality is that two of my current partners have known me for twenty-five years or so, desired me then, and still actively desire me; I've had feedback from other past lovers and friends that I am as desirable, if not more so (I have larger breasts, and a more rounded ass) than I was. The inside of my head doesn't always match the external evidence."

"I lost weight through the depression and anxiety diet after the death of my father. After I had lost 25 pounds, I realized whoa—that is a lot of weight. Maybe I should keep doing this. Part of the problem for me was I wasn't entirely sure what I was doing that was right/correct/good to cause this response in my body. It made me feel different and strange. Yet it also made me feel good. The irony was, of course, I was basically breaking down emotionally, spiritually and as a result I broke down physically as well."

Having complicated feelings about your body and its changes, in turn, can engender complicated feelings about sex. It can be hard, when you're not feeling entirely at home in your body, to feel sexy. If you're not comfortable with a change that has happened with your body, it can be awkward or even painful to have another person praise it or take pleasure from it. It may feel strange or unpleasant to be touched when you don't feel comfortable with a physical change that has taken place. Or you may be okay with being touched but find it difficult or impossible to have an orgasm because part of you is still a bit fixated on whatever's going on with your body change. Sex can tap into some really deep emotions—sometimes things you weren't even aware were going on can come to the surface when sex enters the picture.

Being patient with yourself while you adjust to body change can be hard. It's easy to feel like you should just get over these things or to think that body changes are just physical and therefore superficial. There's nothing superficial about having your body change: your body is you! We all know how stressful it can be to go through changes like switching jobs, moving, planning a wedding, or buying a big-ticket item like a house or a car. Changes to your body aren't any different. If anything, they're even closer to the core of who you are. Don't panic. Give things some time to settle down. And remember: your size and your shape do not define you; they're only a part of the package. You are strong and flexible enough to ride this wave. I promise.

Weight-Loss Dieting and Your Sex Life

At one point or another, for one reason or another, many of us have tried some weight-loss diet or another. Some of us have since given up weight-loss dieting, while others still do it, whether occasionally or frequently.

It's not my aim here to tell anyone what to do or not do as far as their eating habits are concerned. Everyone deserves to eat tasty, nutritious food that they enjoy, as far as I'm concerned, and beyond that it's up to the individual. It is my aim to be honest about how weight-loss dieting specifically may affect your sex life, because you can't make good choices about food or about sex if you don't have good information.

Different people have different experiences with dieting. Some people are able to tolerate it better than others; some find that it doesn't affect their sex drives or experiences one way or another. This varies from person to person, and probably from dietary regime to dietary regime as well, since not all reducing diets are equal in terms of nutrition. That being said, in general, for a large number of people, dieting is likely to be bad for your sex life.

Dieting is stressful. Few people feel sexier or more inclined toward love and sex when they're stressed out. Stressful situations also cause the body's levels of cortisol, a hormone that helps the body cope with stress in the short term, to go up. When stress becomes chronic or ongoing, however, cortisol can contribute to problems that may include elevated blood pressure and blood sugar levels, a weakened immune response, and even damage to the hippocampus region of the brain—not very sexy and more than a little worrisome. Chronic stress can also contribute to anxiety, depression, mood swings, insomnia, and other such unsexy and unhelpful conditions.

"My libido goes way down. I become obsessed with the scale and if I have gained or even stayed the same weight, I get depressed. I start to hate my body because I have a 'goal' to be lighter and I stop being happy just as I am. This spills over into sexuality as well."

Dieting can cause physical symptoms that make people less likely to be interested in sex. Hunger pangs trump desire and so do headaches, constipation, dizziness, irritability, gastrointestinal discomfort, and the like. If you don't feel good, you probably won't feel very sexy or attractive either.

Dieting lowers libido. Loss of libido is a well-documented symptom of starvation. Diets make people lose weight because they are, in effect, a form of controlled semi-starvation where the body is not being given as much fuel as it needs to function, necessitating the use of fat reserves to make up the difference. When your body is experiencing this kind of resource crisis, it tends to reserve its energies for the important task of keeping you alive. Sex is just not as important as survival. Your body doesn't know, and doesn't care, that you are the one limiting its resources and that the limitation is artificial. It will respond as if there is a genuine lack of available nourishment, because, from its perspective, there is.

"This is in the past, but I felt better about myself if I was hungry. I know that's nuts, but it's the truth. I felt I was earning my right to be a sexual being by being hungry. Oh boy. I did not know I felt that until I just wrote it here."

Dieting tends to make one hypercritical of weight, size, and appearance. When you spend a lot of time thinking about what's "wrong" with your body and about your attempt to "fix" it, it's very hard to accept your body as it is, or to accept that someone else might be interested in it. Being able to think only about your physical shortcomings isn't just unsexy for you; it's also unsexy for your partner, who may find your hyperfocus on your body's shortcomings a real buzz kill.

Dieting can be profoundly distracting. Many people who are dieting find that food, eating, weight, weighing, and their diet "progress" occupies a lot of their awareness. No right-thinking individuals want to find themselves wondering whether they can get away with maybe having just the tiniest sliver of a brownie later on, when they're in the middle of kissing someone right now. It's also kind of rude: would you want the person you were making love with to be thinking about how many calories were in that martini he drank at dinner? Or would you prefer him to be thinking about you, and that thing you just did with your tongue?

Dieters can become obsessive, tedious, and boring. We've all had the experience of being around a person who cannot shut up, not even for a second, about a diet. We'd all like to think that this would never be us. But studies have shown that people whose eating is substantially restricted can't necessarily help acting this way: a preoccupation with food is a well-established psychological symptom of starvation. It may not be intentional, but it's still a turnoff.

"I slowly and carefully lost 70 pounds over about a year's time. I felt lighter and stronger, and felt positive about my accomplishment. My overall happiness led to a better quality sex life. I don't believe the body change made much difference, though."

Move It

There are a lot of totally defensible reasons not to like exercise and to not want to do it. It can be hard to tolerate feeling like the embodiment of every sweaty, puffing, fat-person-exercising cliché, among other things. But there is one really excellent reason to strongly consider kicking all that baggage to the curb and moving your body anyway: regular physical movement will, in the vast majority of cases, improve your sex life.

"When I attempt to lose weight, my self-esteem and sex drive nosedive. Once I realized that exercise is awesome even if it doesn't make you lose weight, being more in tune with my body had a positive impact on my sex life."

The reasons for this are mostly simple ones. The body tends to perform best when it gets regular exercise. It evolved to move around a lot, and moving around a lot tends to help keep it functioning right. Joints are stronger and less likely to be injured if the muscles and ligaments that support them are strong and supple. Stamina increases as you build up your physical tolerance for movement. Muscles get stronger when you work them. The heart and lungs get toned and their capacity increases. Your circulation improves, which is really important for sex, since things like erections and orgasms have a lot to do with blood flow and healthy circulation. Improved flexibility will boost your game whether you're at the gym or getting on top. And don't forget that sexual activity is exercise too, and increasing exercise capacity doesn't stop when you cross the bedroom threshold. Increasing your capacity for one kind of exercise will increase your capacity for all the others, including the naked fun kind.

"When I exercise I have more energy for sex, feel more confident in my body, and have more stamina. Sometimes, the positive benefit on my sex life is the major motivator to get me to actually exercise. My wife finds this adorable."

There are other, less physiological reasons that increasing the amount of movement you get can help your sex life. Exercise tends to increase energy levels, something that almost everyone can use. It improves mood as well, with studies showing that it can be as effective as antidepressant drugs in alleviating and preventing depression. Since depression tends to squash the sex drive, this is great news, and even better news considering that lots of antidepressant drugs are also libido flatteners.

The more you move around, the better you get to know your body and the more comfortable you start to feel in your own skin. The more experience you have moving your body around, the more you get to know what it can do, and how far you can trust it. Sure, you may have a tricky knee or a funky elbow (or if you're like me, both), but you get to know them better and at the same time they get stronger, and before too long, you know exactly and intuitively just how much you can do with them without courting injury, either in the gym or in bed. Just between you, me, and the wall, getting regular exercise can make all the difference when it comes to being comfortable getting on top, which is almost enough reason to do it right there. Exercise also helps prevent injuries, whether dur-

"When I started doing Olympic-style weightlifting three years ago (which I LOVE and am still doing) my libido skyrocketed. I have never been this sexually turned on ever."

ing sex or just walking down the street, because your body is stronger and your reflexes are faster.

Exercise isn't just about what you can do physically, though; it's also about spending time genuinely inhabiting your body and feeling connected to it. The more comfortable you get with your body, the easier it is to stay integrated with it, rather than dissociating from it—that "brain in a jar" feeling, where it seems like you are just your consciousness, and your body is a separate thing that isn't really you. Exercising helps you live in your whole body, and be aware of your whole self, which gives you a lot more, literally and figuratively, to bring to sexual experiences. Even if you don't tend to dissociate and have no trouble being present and engaged in your body during sex, the feelings of physical ease and competence that come along with regular movement can add a lot of pleasure and virtuosity to your sexual experience.

"I think exercise can make you more aware of your body and its strength, which is always a positive experience. Like 'Hey—my body can do that! It's pretty cool!' Yoga is great for making you aware of your body, but belly dancing was by far the most positive fat-related exercise I ever did. We worship the belly, the hips, the curves. It makes you feel sooo sexy."

None of this means you have to turn into a gym rat, or that it's all for nothing unless you are exercising for hours every day or become a marathon runner. That's our deeply fascist, totally unrealistic, highly competitive all-or-nothing cult of "the perfect body" talking, not reality, and you should ignore it with extreme prejudice.

What it does mean is that more and more regular movement in your life is good for you and for your sex life. It doesn't really matter what form the movement takes. It could be walking, chair dancing, yoga, cleaning your house, walking your dog, gardening, or anything at all that feels good—or at least neutral—that gets you moving around a bit. In many cases, there are kinds of movement that you can do with

"Being active reminds me that I inhabit this body, and that it is mine—not the other way around. I choose how to use it or not use it, and I can 'fill it out' more as I love it more. I love to dance and to move, and when I am reminded of this by doing it, I feel more sensual."

pleasure even if you have limitations on your mobility. Even a small amount of regular movement can mean a big improvement in your ability to be happier and more confident in your body, and more energetic, enthusiastic, and physically engaged in your sex life. Move it: it makes a difference.

chapter two

Who's Who

Sure, fat people come from all walks of life. But are all fat people alike? Definitely not when it comes to relationships and sex! Find out about the different roles and meanings fatness has for heterosexuals, gays, lesbians, bisexuals, asexuals, kink aficionados, transgender people, fat admirers, and more. Where do you fit in to the big fat picture of sexuality, and who else is out there whom you might like to meet?

Straight but Not Narrow

Numerically speaking, the majority of people identify themselves as heterosexual, and so do the majority of fat people and their partners. At the same time, in our fat-loathing culture it's considered a little odd, a little unusual, a little bit "queer," if you will, for fat people to be sexual at all. For people who are used to thinking of themselves as being sexually "normal" because they identify as heterosexual, this realization can come as a bit of a shock.

In much the same way as gay, lesbian, bisexual, and transgender people have had to learn to do, fat people often have to defend their own sexualities. Our society does not like the idea of fat people having even the most heterosexual sex any more than it likes the idea of any other "deviant" sexual activity. Being straight does not save fat people from having their sexuality mocked, shamed, and used to humiliate and hurt them. You don't have to look any further than the "slap a thigh and ride the wave in" or "pick a fold and fuck it" comments that get made about fat women to see just how pervasive the disgust can be at the idea that fat people are sexual beings at all.

This is why straight fat people can benefit from taking a few pages from the LGBTI movement's playbook. You might not have to come out of the closet about being fat, but you probably will have to come out of the closet as a forthright and unashamed fat person who enjoys a sex life that is very much not a joke. You might not have to defend yourself against gay bashing, but you will probably at some point need to defend yourself or a friend or a lover against fatphobic remarks or cruelty. Just as LGBTI people often have to go to extra effort to get appropriate, respectful sexual health care, so do many fat people. And just as LGBTI people often end up having to justify themselves as human beings deserving of reasonably happy lives even though they do not fit the mainstream ideal, fat people often must do exactly the same.

The LGBTI movement has had great success, and has made great strides in terms of gaining more equality and respect, by refusing to be silent, refusing to be invisible, and refusing to put up with being treated like second-class citizens because their desires and their sexuality happen to make some people uncomfortable. Heterosexual fat people can, and should, do the same. Everybody, and every body, is entitled to dignity and respect, no matter whom they sleep with or what they weigh.

Fat Admirers

Fat admirers. Chubby chasers. Plumper humpers. You can call 'em what you like, but they all have one thing in common: they like fat. They gravitate toward partners whose bodies are anything but the mainstream thin-is-in ideal. They like the roundness and heaviness and fullness of fat bodies, the curve and the roll of them, the heft and the sturdiness, the softness and the generosity and the warmth. There are male fat admirers and female and trans, straight and queer and bisexual. They come in all colors, from all places, and from all different kinds of backgrounds. Although *fat admirer* and *FA* are most often used to refer to heterosexual men who are interested in fat women, *fat admirer* as a phrase describes anyone who has a sexual or romantic interest in fat partner(s).

Not all fat admirers like the same exact things. It makes sense: people who are attracted to thinner people aren't necessarily attracted to every thin person they see, either. People have their special likes and their particular quirks. Some fat admirers are most attracted to fat bodies that are on the fattest end of the fat spectrum, preferring supersized bodies over any others. But other fat admirers might prefer people who are sort of medium fat or maybe even bodies that some people would say were merely on the large end of average.

The same diversity exists in terms of liking different body shapes and types. There are diehard belly fans and equally fervent devotees of big butts and thighs. Big breasts in women are a favorite for lots of people, but not everyone who is attracted to fat women is automatically a breast fan. In some cases, fat admirers are open to a wide variety of body shapes and sizes and types. In other cases, only one very specific body shape or type will trip their trigger.

This might seem disheartening if you're a fat person. If fat admirers' tastes are so specific, what are the chances that any given fat person, namely you, will fill the bill? It may seem like yet again, the odds are against you. In reality, this hasn't got anything to do with you. Nor does it affect your odds of finding a partner who is into exactly what you are. All it means is that fat admirers are no different from anyone else. Liking fat bodies doesn't mean you necessarily like all fat bodies, or even all fat people who have the particular type of fat body you prefer. Fat or thin, attraction still depends an awful lot on some very personal and subjective chemistry.

Fat admirers have their own particular set of issues that are covered in more detail in chapter 4, For Fat Admirers Only (page 111). Many fat admirers struggle with being closeted about their attractions as do their fat partners who have to deal with the fallout of closeting. These partners may end up feeling like their partners consider them good enough for sex but not good enough for more full-fledged relationships or for sharing a life. Fat admirer culture and the different roles that fat admirers can play in the lives of fat people are also issues that have specific resonance.

It's worth noting that not every fat admirer has always been a fat admirer, and not all fat admirers will be attracted to fat people all the time or every time. Some fat admirers know they are fat admirers from the earliest moments that they are aware of having romantic and sexual interests. Other people come to it later in life. Still others are not fat admirers in any general sense of the term but are absolutely 100 percent smitten by one particular fat person and completely thrilled by that person's body and appearance along with everything else. Some fat admirers, although certainly not all of them, are specifically sexually aroused by fatness itself, or by the particular visual and sensory stimulation that fat can provide. Some of these people might consider themselves fat fetishists, although others may not. (See "Fat as Fetish," page 189.)

Fat-admirer issues apply to all of these people. Anyone who likes, desires, and appreciates fat partners, whether once or consistently throughout their lifetime, is engaging in fat admiration. Being a fat admirer is not limited to the relatively small number of people who self-label that way. In fact, it's quite a bit more common than you may think.

Fat people and fat admirers alike should bear in mind that a liking for bigger bodies is not the same thing as being open minded, accepting, and tolerant of difference across the board. It is easy to fall into the trap of thinking that since fat admirers are open to something so far removed from the mainstream, namely finding fat bodies attractive, they must be just as free thinking and groovy about other kinds of nonmainstream personal differences. Alas, this is not the case. It is quite possible to not participate in mainstream prejudices on the issue of fatness while still participating in others. Fat admirers can still be prejudiced about, and discriminate against, people on the basis of disability, age, race, class, looks, and all manner of other things. One could wish it were otherwise, but this too is merely more evidence that desiring fat people is really not so different than desiring any other kind of people. Desire is one thing, and political principles are typically another.

Fat Asexuals: Probably Not What You're Thinking

Asexuality has only recently started to be recognized as a genuine, valid manifestation of human sexuality. This is long overdue. Not everybody is interested in sex in the same ways. Some people aren't interested in sex at all. Others don't experience strong sexual or romantic attraction to anyone; yet other people experience romantic attraction but not sexual desire. Other people experience these things only once or twice and otherwise don't feel the pull. For some people a lack of interest in sex and/or romance is something that comes and goes. Any of this, and all of this, can be perfectly normal, healthy, and okay. Asexuality is just another place on the spectrum of sexual and romantic interest and desire.

People who identify themselves as asexual come in all shapes, sizes, colors, sexes, and types. They do not share any common history. They do not all feel or think the same way about their asexuality. All they have in common is that they don't have the same degree or kind of interest in many or any of the kinds of sexual and sexual-romantic relationships that tend to be of so much interest to other people.

Fat people who are asexual may seem, to some people, to be the living embodiment of a fat-hating cliché. Because fat people are so often perceived and portrayed as being people who *should not* be sexual, or for whom sexuality is inappropriate, actually being fat and asexual comes with a whole array of stereotypes that can make it hard to feel positive or even neutral about one's asexuality. There is a whole train of anti-fat psychoanalytical thought that claims that fat people are fat because they are hiding from their sexuality, as if being fat would automatically put all sexual concerns on hold. Being fat doesn't do this, first of all. (If it did, there'd be no point to this book!) Second, having confronted and identified one's asexuality is not the same thing as being afraid of one's sexuality or hiding from it.

One asexual woman interviewed for this book spoke directly to this cliché. "The classic psychoanalytic interpretation is that fat is a barrier to intimacy. But I know this to be nonsense: the only times I want to be 'intimate' (in a loving, but nonsexual, way) are when I'm overweight. If the weight were a barrier, it would logically follow that when you removed it, you would want the intimacy. In fact, the exact opposite is true: when I diet and lose a lot of weight, I become completely ascetic and solitary, not desiring human contact at all. I only feel 'sexy,' or have any hormonal urges, when I'm overweight. When I lose weight, all of the sensualities (like food and sex) are eradicated simultaneously."

Another asexually identifying woman agreed: "When we're talking about negative responses to asexuality, there are two common appearance-related ones: 'You're asexual because you can't get laid' and 'Since you *could* get laid, you can't be asexual.' I've been told the second one and even though it seems more complimentary, and people might mean it as a good thing, it's equally insulting because it's a total denial of my identity." So much for the stereotypes!

Another common stereotype about asexuality and fatness is that asexuals must have an easier time with self-acceptance and with having a positive body image because they don't have to worry about sex or whether or not other people find them sexually desirable. This is not necessarily the case. "I have had asexual relationships and still have issues with body acceptance [of myself]," a third asexually identified interviewee said. "This is due to a variety of factors (childhood, environment, media, self-esteem), but asexuality is not one of them. . . . Why would my not having expectations of sex have anything to do with how fat I am, or how pretty I look?"

Asexuals, in other words, may face as wide and varied an array of issues relating to size, weight, and sex as everybody else. Asexuality does not, in fact, simplify the complicated landscape of size and sexuality. We can't jump to conclusions about asexuality on the basis of a person's weight or size, and we certainly can't jump to conclusions about weight or size on the basis of a person's asexuality. Even the "fat acceptance" movement should take care, in its efforts to help fat people reclaim their sexual autonomy, not to assume that everyone is sexual. "What I hear a lot in the fat acceptance community is stuff like, 'Fat people have been desexualized, but actually we are sexual beings,'" one woman said. "That kind of thing is frustrating because 99 percent of [fat people] may be sexual beings, but that's no reason to erase the 1 percent (at least) who aren't."

Chubbies and Chasers and Bears, Oh My!

Gay and bisexual men are legendary for forming sexuality-based communities, and fat-related sexuality has been no exception. Although the body standards of mainstream gay male culture can at times be so narrow and exacting as to border on the fascistic, and many gay men are primarily or exclusively attracted to "thin and beautiful" men, queer men's tastes and desires run the same wide gamut as anybody else's. Men who celebrate and enjoy fat men are just as likely to be vocal, visible, and proud as any other queer guys.

Across North America and around the world, there are chapters of an organization called Girth and Mirth, a social club for fat gay men and the men who are attracted to them. Gay fat admirers are usually called *chasers* or *chub chasers*, and fat gay men are called *chubs*. Girth and Mirth chapters hold get-togethers at restaurants and bars, are a presence in Pride parades and community organizing, do work to benefit charities, hold parties for their members, and participate in regional, national, and even international conferences. Girth and Mirth chapters can be located by looking for listings in local and regional gay community newspapers, by calling local gay community centers, and by searching for "Girth and Mirth" online. Associated Big Men's Clubs is an umbrella organization that includes numerous chub/chaser organizations.

Gay male culture also encompasses the "bear" subculture, which also includes a large number of fat men and guys who are attracted to them. There is some overlap between *bear* and *chub*. Bears tend to be hairy, in terms of both facial hair and body hair, and may dress and groom themselves in a style that is very traditionally masculine and rugged. Chubs may or may not be hairy,

"Finding my local Girth and Mirth was a great thing for me. Learning that there were guys who totally loved my body made up for a lot of the really nasty vicious bullshit I had experienced at clubs. I would recommend Girth and Mirth to any fat gay man, especially if he's just coming out. It's really nice to get to know other guys who deal with the same issues. And of course the guys who think you're hot."

and their dress and other aspects of their gender vary more widely. More to the point, not all bears are fat, while fatness is a defining characteristic of chubs. Not all chubs are bears, but some bears are definitely chubs.

Bears also have their own distinctive subculture. There are "bear bars" and bear social groups, bear clubs, and bear events including weekends, conferences, and even chartered cruise ship journeys just for bears and bear lovers.

In addition to social opportunities and community building, there are many other resources available to the fat gay/bi man and those who desire him. Bear- and chub-themed books and media, including plenty of pornography, are available online and at many LGBTI bookstores.

Looksism can still be a major issue in chub/chaser and bear culture, and so can sizeism. A handsome face still counts for a great deal, as do grooming, clothes, and whether or not a man fits in well with the aesthetic standards of his particular community: a bear with a badly kept beard may be a lonely one. As for body sizes, tastes differ just as they do among other fat admirers. Some men prefer bears who are not so much fat as burly and muscular; others seek out the big hairy bellies like homing beacons. As in other orientational demographics, knowing that someone is a fat admirer does not necessarily tell you everything there is to know about what he specifically likes.

Glorious Dykes

Lesbian culture has long been a highly political culture, and queer women of all stripes have a long and well-deserved reputation as political and social firebrands of extraordinary capability, strength, and persistence. This is also true when it comes to fat issues. Much that is central to body-acceptance politics, art, and social organizing has had roots in the queer women's community, and some of the most exciting fat-acceptance work going on today is also based there.

This is not to say that the queer women's community is a magic fat utopia where everyone is universally accepting. Individual queer women, including fat queer women, may carry around hefty amounts of anti-fat prejudice. In the queer women's community, as everywhere, fatness can be controversial and is sometimes reviled. However, the influence of feminist politics on the queer women's community means that women are less likely, overall, to be judged overtly for their appearance than they are in mainstream heterosexually oriented culture. For political reasons, standards of politeness and civility in queer women's spaces generally include at least public (if not always private) tolerance of all women's bodies and a general philosophical agreement that women do not have to conform to mainstream beauty standards to be beautiful and desirable. It may not be utopia, but it's certainly a far cry from mainstream culture's take on these issues.

Perhaps the biggest jewel in the crown of queer women's current organizing and political work around fatness is the organization NOLOSE, the National Organization of Lesbians of SizE. NOLOSE is a volunteer-run organization that is "dedicated to ending the oppression of fat people and creating vibrant fat queer culture." It includes a wide range of women and trans-identified people who are fat or who are allies of fat queer women and trans-identified people. NOLOSE's conferences are a highlight of the radical political scene, and many attendees find the experience transformative, both personally and politically. For more information about NOLOSE, see the Resource Guide.

Some urban areas also have social groups and/or events centering on fat queer women, including clothing swaps or clothes recycling events like the Fat Girl Flea Market that takes place yearly in New York City. These are sometimes word-of-mouth affairs, but they may also be listed in area LGBTI newspapers, or information may be available from gay community centers. If there is no queer fat women's group where you are, or simply no fat women's group (most, whether they originate in the queer movement or not, are welcoming to all women), you might consider starting one. Fat-accepting women's culture is and always has been very much a DIY phenomenon, and grassroots activity is central to its existence and its success.

Oh, and since we're on the subject, no, fat women don't become lesbians because they are too fat to get men. Fat women who want to have sex or relationships with men can generally find men willing to oblige them. Fat women who are lesbians are generally lesbians for the same reason any thinner lesbian is a lesbian: they are sexually attracted by and emotionally drawn to other women. Weight has nothing to do with this.

Some lesbians report that they feel more accepting of their own fatness because they feel that heterosexual mainstream ideals about beauty and body size are simply irrelevant to their lives. Others don't feel any less body size or weight pressure from mainstream culture just because they are queer. Not every fat queer woman will have the same experience.

Bi and Large

Yes, Virginia, there are fat bisexuals, just as there are fat gay men, lesbians, transgender folks, asexuals, and oh, yes, straight people. Unfortunately, however, bisexuals have yet to succeed in forming the same kind of extensive community around sexuality that other queer cultures have produced. (This is not, I must note, for lack of trying. Many bisexual activists, some of whom are fat, continue to fight that good fight.) Fat bisexuals can thus be found everywhere fat people exist—in straight, gay, trans, lesbian, queer, kinky, celibate, and every other kind of milieu.

Fatness does not make people bisexual. Occasionally, you will run across a person who is convinced that a fat bisexual became bisexual because fatness ruined his or her chances with the opposite sex so the person decided to turn to same-sex partners instead. In reality bisexual people are bisexual because they're attracted to and sexually interested in more than just one sex, something that has nothing to do with fatness.

Trans Fats

Transgender people come in all shapes and sizes, just like everyone else. Fatness can be an asset to some trans people and can pose a hurdle for others. But whether and how it is an asset can depend quite a bit on what sort of trans person one is, is expected to be, or aspires to become.

Male-to-female trans people, like biological women generally, often find that fatness is more of a burden than it is a blessing. Depending on where a trans woman carries her fat, and whether it is firm or squishy, she may be able to use her fat to produce more feminine body shape and curves. The right foundation garments can help a lot with this. If a trans woman carries her fat in the male-typical "apple" pattern, however, it can make a traditionally feminine body shape more difficult to achieve.

Some trans women, especially those who are heterosexually identified, may be very invested in achieving mainstream ideals of feminine beauty, including a thin body. The thin mainstream beauty ideal can also become an issue in medical care. Doctors who manage trans women's hormonal and other medical maintenance often hold their patients to a strict and narrow definition of what acceptable femininity should look like; some trans women have experienced doctors threatening to withhold hormone prescriptions until weight loss occurs. Doctors may claim that a trans woman's failure to toe the line of the thin-centric female beauty ideal means that she is not really serious about being a woman. (One wonders whether they also believe that genetic females who are fat are likewise not really serious about being women.) Or they may contend that there are too many health risks for fat people to take estrogen. (Oddly, genetic females who are fat manage to get along just fine with both fat and estrogen in their bodies.) Healthy women's bodies can exist in a full range of types and sizes and shapes, and transgender women are no different.

Female-to-male trans people, like biological men generally, often find that they can get away with greater amounts of fatness without taking too much guff for it. Fat can, in fact, help produce a more believably masculine body shape. Trans men who naturally carry their weight in the male-typical "apple" pattern have a built-in boost to their gender presentation. Trans men whose bodies naturally store fat in other places, such as breasts and hips, can use binders (undergarments with heavy elastic) to smooth out the curves into something more burly than curvy, although just as with born-male people, pear-shaped bodies can still suggest a certain femininity that may not be welcome.

Again, though, the boost to gender presentation provided by fatness can be a double-edged sword. Gay-identified trans men, depending on the types of men and gay male subcultures they are interested in, may or may not find that fatness helps their case. For trans men who are interested in chub/chaser or bear dynamics, fatness would not be much of a liability, but for trans men who are more interested in, for example, the dance club scene, it may make fitting in more difficult.

Fat and Kinky

The definition of *kinky* can depend a lot on the person using the word. Human beings have an almost infinite variety of sexual variety at their disposal, and the reasons that some things are labeled "kinky" and other things designated "vanilla" are complicated, subjective, and not entirely devoid of controversy. Is it kinky for a woman to be sexually submissive to her male partner? Or is that just an expression of normative sexual roles? (And is a normative sex role structure that historically requires the submission of one group of people and their domination by another kinky all by itself? People have been fighting over this one for decades.) We could just as easily ask if it is kinky to desire a fat partner. Certainly it is typically seen, especially in the pornography industry, as a specialized taste, sometimes as a fetish. To call it a *kink*, though, would certainly be controversial to many people.

For most purposes, the word *kinky* is a stand-in for a collection of what psychiatry has historically called *paraphilias*—erotic interests in things that are not part of genitally oriented sex. The kinky spectrum includes fetishes for body parts or inanimate objects, interest in particular types of sensations (including pain), interest in particular emotional or psychological states, interest in certain social power dynamics, and much else. BDSM (Bondage/Discipline/Dominance/ Submission/Sadism/Masochism) is part of what falls under the kinky umbrella, but so do many other things. It's commonly considered kinky to find latex clothing erotic or to get sexual satisfaction from being tickled.

Large and extensive communities of people with interests in kink exist both online and off. Some kinky communities are specifically oriented toward people who are heterosexually identified, some to people who are LGBTI-identified, and some are open to anyone regardless of how they identify in terms of sexual orientation. Fat people may be part of any of these.

Many people have noticed that it sometimes seems as if there are far more fat than thin people in kinky communities. This is often attributed to the fact that kinky sexuality often has different priorities and aesthetics than mainstream "vanilla" sexuality. Where mainstream sexuality might be all about conforming to a Hollywood beauty ideal or how many porn-star positions someone can manage, kinky sexuality might focus on the physical strength and imposing size of a dominant or the pleasing way that a big soft rear end offers a fantastic surface for paddling. In kinky communities, too, chemistry between potential partners can have a lot more to do with compatible tastes in kink than it does with more superficial factors like pants size.

Occasionally, one encounters situations where kink-like power dynamics are brought into play specifically with regard to weight gain or weight loss. If one partner demands that the other partner either lose or gain weight, this should set off special alarm bells in your head: only the person whose body it is should be making decisions about changing that body. No one else gets to be the boss of your body but you. If someone else is insisting or demanding that you change your body shape or size for that person's pleasure, or hinting that if you really loved them you would do this or that thing to your body, do not hesitate to say no or even to leave the relationship if necessary. This is a situation with an enormous potential for abuse.

This is also true of any activity that someone else asks you to do or wants to do to you but to which you cannot give your informed and enthusiastic consent. Being kinky does not mean that you have to do everything that some other kinky person asks. Even if you identify as a "submissive" or a "slave," you are entitled to your own boundaries about what is and isn't okay for you. Kink is negotiated, self-aware, respectful of boundaries, and mutually consensual. Abuse is not. If it feels like abuse, it probably is. (For more on various forms of kink, see "BDSM," page 185; "Fat as Fetish," page 189; and "Feederism," page 192.)

chapter three

Getting a Grip

Many of the most difficult obstacles in our pursuit of happy, healthy, and abundant love and sex lives are the emotional and psychological ones. Living in a culture that despises fatness means that merely learning to like and love ourselves without shame can be hard work. Yet this is precisely what we have to do in order to be open to the kinds of excitement, pleasure, and big sustaining loves that we want in our lives. This section covers many parts of the ongoing project of defining and developing yourself as a sexy, vital, desiring, and desired human being, including learning to like what you see in the mirror, coping with both positive and negative attention, being more comfortable getting naked in front of other people, and making peace with your belly. . . and maybe even with your mom.

Changing What You See

The biggest and most difficult problem fat people encounter with regard to sexuality really has very little to do with sex itself. It doesn't have anything to do with finding other people who think they are attractive or desirable, either. The biggest and most difficult problems fat people encounter with regard to sex are (1) believing that they are desirable and (2) getting over body related shame.

"Can we erase the shame that kills the libido sometimes? 'Cause seriously. You're amazing."

When you are ashamed of your body and don't believe that you're desirable, a thousand people can be clamoring for your attentions and you still won't buy it. When you've convinced yourself that you're not anything anyone else would want, you won't feel sexy, you won't feel cute, and you won't feel handsome or sassy or confident. You probably won't take a chance on flirting, let alone making a pass at someone, if you're convinced that they couldn't possibly be interested. When you're stuck in your own little world of unlovability and undesirability, you might not even be able to take someone seriously when they tell you flat out that they're interested.

So how do you learn to believe that you really are desirable? How can you rewire your thought processes so that you are able to see yourself as someone who is interesting, attractive, cute, sexy, and well worth anybody's attention?

There's no quick fix. You didn't learn to hate fat bodies in a single day or a single year. It took growing up and spending many years in a society in which fat bodies are considered the legitimate subjects of all kinds of mockery and abuse, to internalize the idea that because you are fat, it is absolutely impossible that anyone could find you desirable. We live in a culture where even celebrities who are conventionally beautiful, thin, toned, rich, and admired often think of themselves as ugly ducklings whose success could vanish overnight if they don't stick to rigorous, constant diet and exercise regimes to try to toe the line and continue to "look good enough."

This isn't false modesty on their part, really. It's the result of a culture where no body is ever good enough, ever pretty

"Twice I've had guys tell me they were interested in me and wanted to go out and I basically just said no and then avoided them. I was convinced they were lying or maybe trying to set me up as a joke, ha ha, it's so funny when the fat girl thinks you're into her, ha ha, or that they thought I'd be desperate and easy. Found out later that one of them at least was really upset and really did have a thing for me. I have to say I still don't really understand why."

enough, ever thin or toned or perfect enough. It's the product of a society where just about the worst thing you can say about anyone and the insult most likely to get straight under someone's skin, particularly if they're female, is to call that person "fat." This is what teaches fat people to despise themselves to the point that they can't even admit that someone else might find them desirable. And it takes some time and effort to even begin to undo it.

> "The single best thing I did in terms of learning to accept my own body for what it is was to stop watching television. Kill your TV! You'll be surprised how much free time you have, and also how much less toxic imagery is filling up your head and making you think less of yourself."

Learning to accept yourself, and to understand that you too can be desirable, starts with learning to expand your horizons. Changing what you see when you see other fat people is a great way to start changing what you see when you look in the mirror. When you are able to see what might be attractive about other people whose bodies are more like yours than they are like, say, Halle Berry's, your chances of being able to see what others might find desirable about yours are vastly increased.

As an exercise, try finding something to compliment in every fat person you see. You don't have to actually pay the compliment, of course, although you can, and it's a great thing to do. Perhaps you see a fat woman with beautiful skin or a wonderful fashion sense. Maybe you notice a fat man who carries himself with grace or whose eyes have a sparkly glint that's irresistible. Check out those powerful calves on that dude over there! Look at how sassy that big girl over there looks in that skinny little pencil skirt! There is almost always something that you can, with complete honesty, see as appealing.

Another thing that can be useful in helping you change the way you see fat bodies, says health counselor Golda Poretsky, is to start really paying attention when you look around you. "Part of the struggle with believing that someone else finds you attractive is that we get conditioned by advertising, other forms of media, and often by people in our lives that in order to be attractive you need to be thin, or at least thinner. But when you actually look at the people around you, you start to notice a different reality. Most of us know fat people who are in great relationships. We also know fat people in less great relationships and who are single. We also know thin people who are single and in not-so-great relationships and in great relationships. In other words, when you look at people you actually know and their dating lives, you can start to let go of some of the assumptions about size and attractiveness." This makes sense. When you let yourself notice the genuine variety of what's actually out there, the stereotype and media version of what's supposedly "real" and "true" increasingly gets cut down to size.

"I believe growing up morbidly obese allowed me the opportunity to be completely divorced from our culture's standards of beauty, so I could make my own. I could decide that I'm beautiful as I am, without much pressure to change one thing or another (since it would take SO much change to fit in!). I came to value authenticity above cultural norms, and that has led me to amazing relationships and an amazing sex life. I'm certain there are other paths to those values, but this one was my path."

Fake It 'Til You Make It

The best advice I ever got about how to succeed—at pretty much anything in the social arena—was "Fake it 'til you make it." I know some people think it's putting the cart before the horse—that if you don't genuinely have or feel whatever it is, no amount of faking it will help the situation. And this might well be true if what you're trying to fake is, let's say, performing surgery, juggling chainsaws, or playing a piano concerto. When it comes to self-confidence and a good sexy self-image, on the other hand, faking it 'til you make it not only helps, but it can actually create the very thing you're trying to emulate.

In social situations, and particularly with new people, you want to be the very best version of yourself that you can. The very best version of yourself is, without question, a confident one—not arrogant, not conceited, not pushy, just confident: confident that you can go

continued on page 79

INTERVIEW:
Seeing Your Attractiveness More Clearly with Golda Poretsky

Golda Poretsky is a New York City–based health counselor with a background in integrative nutrition who decided to stop dieting—permanently—in 2007. Since then, through her company Body Love Wellness, she has been counseling people of all sizes and sexes on how to develop more self-loving, self-nurturing, and happier relationships with their bodies, in workshops, one-on-one counseling, and phone counseling.

Q: *Even the most body-loving of us sometimes has bad days. How do you help people cope with it when they're having a serious Ugly Fit?*

A: A big part of accepting and loving yourself and your body is accepting the fact that you're not always going to feel 100 percent fabulous and making sure to accept and love yourself up when it does happen. One of the best things to do is to treat yourself as if you're a researcher of your own life. Notice the people and situations that trigger Ugly Fits, whether it's being reviewed at work, having to wear a bridesmaid dress, or particular relatives or friends. Then when that negative voice creeps up, you can tell yourself, "Oh, I'm feeling this way because this is the way I always feel when [thing] happens." You can also remind yourself that when that negative voice shows up, you don't have to agree with it and let it bring you down. Acknowledge its presence and remind yourself that it's not the truth.

Q: *What are some good strategies for regrouping and recuperating after your ability to accept your own attractiveness has taken a hit—after you've gotten insulted on the street or your mother has nagged you about how much nicer you'd look if you could wear that in a smaller size, or whatever?*

A: I could give a bunch of tips here, but there's a bigger point I'd like to make. Here's the thing about deciding to love your body and feel attractive no matter what—it's a completely revolutionary act. You are constantly in opposition to a system of oppression that has infiltrated every aspect of society, and, as such, the path you've chosen is not easy. You are going to face people and situations all the time that challenge your truth and your path. And you have to decide in those moments and after those moments, "Do I want to give my power up to this status quo of oppression, or do I keep fighting?"

That doesn't mean that you always have to have a snappy comeback when you get insulted on the street, or fight with your mom all the time about your size, but it does mean that you have to move through your life acknowledging your self-worth, your beauty, and your power. Know that you are a revolutionary, you are fighting the power, you are changing society by not giving in to all of its rules, and you are bringing along others with your example, whether you are always aware of it or not. It's not comfortable to be a revolutionary, but it's also where the biggest rewards are. So when you have these moments where your attractiveness takes a hit, take back your power by acknowledging the fact that you are a hot, sexy, body-loving revolutionary.

continued

Q: *If you could wave your magic wand and have every fat person in America do three things to help their ability to see and understand their own attractiveness and desirability, what would those three things be?*

A: I love this question. Though it's hard to pick only three, I would say (1) have weekly self-care rituals that you enjoy, (2) make sure to wear clothes that you like, and (3) use affirmations or mantras that turn you on and make you feel good when you say them or think them.

The first one, self-care rituals, is really about putting the attention on yourself and doing something just because it gives you pleasure. Self-care rituals can be anything from taking a candlelit bath with your favorite music playing to taking a dance class to playing with your dog. By consistently making time for yourself, putting yourself first, and connecting with your pleasure, you naturally become more alive and more attractive to others.

Second, wearing clothes that you like is so important. As fat people, we get a weird mixed message around shopping. Many of us feel like we should wear clothes that hide and cover our bodies and buy clothes that are too small, to encourage us to stick to a diet. This is just insanity! You've got to let go of the clothes that are way too small as well as the clothes that make you feel dumpy. Experiment and have fun with dressing the body that you have right now.

Third, using affirmations is hugely helpful. I know it sounds goofy, and I've had a lot of clients who were resistant to the idea, but once they started using affirmations it had a really powerful impact on their ability to see their attractiveness. Start with a really simple one, like "I'm attractive" or "I'm beautiful." Think it when you're walking down the street. Write it out in a journal. Say it in front of a mirror. You may have lots of resistance and it may even seem like a huge lie, but as you keep reinforcing this truth, you will begin to feel it within.

In your opinion, what are the best things about sexuality as a fat person?

"Cuddliness. I'm so lovely and soft, I like to cuddle myself."

"I love my soft belly, my hips and my solid thighs. I love lying on my back and feeling the way my breasts sort of fall to the side, the curve as my chest flattens down and bulges at the side. That to me is fantastically sexy. And of course I love having sex with fat men!"

"My BOUNDLESS, rugby-team-beating, willing-to-take-on-a-whole-flock-of-Dykes-on-Bikes sexual appetite."

"Surprising people when they realize I'm not ashamed of my body."

"We are just so opulent, aren't we? I mean we are all curves, all softness. I have super silky skin and that is great for sex. Also, more surface area means more areas to touch. I think the wonderful thing about being fat is that it has made me really confront my body and my sexuality. Being so comfortable with who I am makes sex great."

"NOT worrying about the ways in which my body moves—my fat has a life of its own, and the movements of sex are echoed in the movement of my fat!"

"My partner and I, both fat, are honest and caring and frank with one another. We laugh all the time, and enjoy the hell out of each other. That's the best thing—both in bed and out."

"We are fucking good in bed."

"My softness by far. I am also married to a man who loves every inch of me. I can be totally naked and bending over to pick up socks, and he thinks I am hot. It feels amazing. So—during sex, I get all naked, leave the lights on and leave any inhibitions on the floor with my panties."

continued

"I have lots of flesh and skin, which means lots of sensation pleasure. I like the feeling of my flesh and skin sliding against a partner's and the thud of our bodies together, resounding in the room and through my body."

"I've been a thin person and a fat person. The sex I had when I was thin was certainly more athletic, but I was also having it with clueless fumbling college boys. The sex I have when I'm fat (and both my partners are large men) is more meandering and sensual. It's less goal-oriented. 'Let's stay in bed all day.' My partners know what they like and what the hell they're doing, and I know what I like and what I'm doing. I don't know if that's a specific advantage of fat, but it is an advantage of age and increased confidence."

"I didn't grow up fat, but thin does not equal pretty. I had zits, perms, glasses, horrific orthodontia, and zero social skills or fashion sense as a kid. The thing I had going for me was intelligence. I got rewarded for being smart. It freed me from a lot of the oppression that women and girls get around their looks."

"Oddly enough, I grew more confident as I grew in size, because once I passed a certain weight I didn't waste any more time debating whether or not to take off my shirt for fear that my partner would notice the rolls of fat on my belly. After I gained weight, the rolls of fat were visible whether I was wearing clothes or not, so I no longer feared that the person I was flirting with had mistaken me for someone with a lingerie-model's body, only to be disappointed when I stripped. I never worried about 'do I look fat in this position?' as some of my slender friends had worried, because of course I did! I felt free from worry!"

"Having never really fit the cultural ideal, what physical enjoyment I experience has already been fought for and won. Some battles are behind me that other women my age have yet to face."

after what you want, confident that there's a good chance you might get it, confident that if you don't get it after all you'll still be just fine. People who exude that sort of confidence are pleasant and encouraging to be around. The attitude is likeable and contagious and very attractive. You know how with some people, it's hard to know whether you want them or you want to be them or maybe both? Confidence is a big part of what provokes that sort of reaction.

Acting as if you really can go after what you want, secure in the knowledge that you have as good a chance as anyone and will be just fine whatever happens, goes a long way. It's what's called a self-fulfilling prophecy. It won't necessarily give you the Midas touch. Nor will it instantly change everything about the way you think and feel about yourself, or even just about risk taking. Over time, though, it makes a pretty significant dent.

One of the things that you learn when you take the "fake it 'til you make it" path is that real disaster happens a lot less often than you might fear. Most of the time, if you go into a situation assuming that you'll be just fine no matter what happens, you really will. Similarly, if you go into a situation with the attitude that there's no real reason that your size or weight should be an impediment to having a good time or meeting someone interesting or leaving with the phone number of that cutie you met last week, chances are better than average that you'll be absolutely right.

If "fake it 'til you make it" seems too, well, fake, here's another way to think about the same general thing: think of it in terms of acting like the kind of person you want to be when you grow up. We all have an ideal in our heads of the kind of competent, high-functioning person we'd like to be, the kind of smart, effective person we imagine we would really enjoy being. Sometimes we think of this ideal self as what we'd be like if only we were thin: "I'd be more like that if I lost the weight." And that's the whole point: you don't have to wait. You don't have to wait until you grow up, you don't have to wait until you lose weight, you don't have to wait until there's an out lesbian in the Oval Office. There's nothing stopping you from being more like who you are, or who you want to be, this very minute.

So what would the person you want to be when you grow up be thinking as he went into a social situation? How would he approach an attractive stranger? What would she say if someone interesting asked for a phone number or for a date or a hookup? How would that person deal with a "thanks, but no thanks" from someone he had approached? How would she explain to a sex partner exactly how she liked to be touched? If you can figure this out, you don't have to wait: you can start doing it now.

Sometimes this approach will work better than others. Sometimes it will feel more organic and natural than others. This is normal and totally to be expected. Keep working toward being your best version of yourself, and in time you will begin to realize that your best self is, after all, just part of your real self, and that you do have a bountiful personal supply of exactly the kind of confidence and competence that will always stand you in good stead. It doesn't matter what you weigh, it doesn't matter what you wear: it's yours, and all you have to do is make it so.

Tell Me What You Want

As a result of our fat-hating culture, fat people often grow up with the belief that their sexual and romantic desires don't really matter because they're fat. Beggars can't be choosers, we're told. Only beautiful, thin, conventionally attractive people get to have exactly what they want in love and romance. Fat people have to make do with what they can get.

How lovely to know that this isn't true! Getting what one wants in love and sex is not a cosmic reward that is bestowed upon people when they have finally achieved "The Correct Body." In real life, sex and love lives happen to people with all kinds of bodies. They are usually an untidy—but potentially highly satisfying—mixture of what people want, what's available to choose from, and what they and their partner(s) can create together.

Knowing what you want is part of the process of getting it, or at least getting something close enough to be satisfying. You don't have to specify a lot of details; in fact, too many details and specifics can be more of a hindrance than a help. But general parameters are great. Do you want a casual relationship or a serious one? Do you want a relationship that includes sex right from the start or one where sex will come into the picture only when you feel emotionally committed to one another? Do you like a relationship with a sizeable friendship component or do you believe that sexual relationships and friendships shouldn't mix? It's good, and very useful, to know where you stand and what you're looking for.

Sometimes it helps to think about this question in terms of what you *don't* want. You may not know yet whether you want a casual relationship or a serious one, but if you know that you definitely don't want a relationship with someone who is rebounding from a previous relationship, that certainly helps narrow the field and puts a useful boundary into place. You might not know whether you're going to want a relationship to be sexual right from the start or whether you're going to want to wait a little, but you may know that you are not interested in a relationship with someone who doesn't share your political beliefs. This is one of the places where prior relationships—even the serious crash-and-burn ones—come in really handy. As an old teacher of mine used to say, "No one is useless; they can always serve as a bad example." The bad examples in your past can also make up part of a useful checklist of "don't wants" for your future.

You'll notice that there are some kinds of things I haven't suggested as "things to want," like hair color, height, weight, or other appearance-related things. That's because although we all have our preferences for appearances and style and so on, good love, good sex, and great relationships can look like a lot of things. Have all the preferences you like, but remember that there is also a very real possibility that excellent relationships and fantastic sex partners may come in physical packages that are not necessarily exactly like your fantasy ideal. Sometimes looks and style and similar factors can be legitimate deal breakers, and there's nothing wrong with that. But it can also be a little too easy, sometimes, to throw the baby out with the bathwater. You can't tell a book by its cover, and sometimes the perfect person shows up wearing a face or a body that you wouldn't initially imagine contains the fantastic human being it does. You don't have to settle for anything that is unacceptable to you, but, on the other hand, if it can work to your advantage to be flexible, why not at least give it a try?

The same thing is true of desires that are specifically about sexual activity. As difficult as it can be to be clear about what you want with regard to relationships, it can be at least as difficult to be clear about what you want sexually. Sometimes people feel dirty or embarrassed even saying the words, and they really have to work hard to be able to say things like "I like it when someone nibbles on the insides of my thighs" or even "Oooh, that feels sensational—do that again."

It can be challenging to verbalize your desires at that very vulnerable intersection of your body, desires, and physical sensation. Some people find it useful to practice with something less highly charged, like a backrub or back scratch. A good exercise is to make an agreement with the person rubbing or scratching that they will do only what you direct them to do, so that you have to give a continuous stream of directions and feedback. It might seem awkward at first, but after even just a few minutes, it gets easier. You quickly learn that general instructions like "Okay, scratch my back" aren't so useful to your partner or to you, while more detailed instructions like "Up and to the right about three inches; yes, right there, harder!" give your partner a lot more information and you a lot more of what you're looking for. Later on, try transferring the same principle, or even the same exercise, to something more explicitly sexual, like a hand job or finger fucking. It's really not so different.

A key element to all of this is trust. It can be hard to expose your vulnerable desires—and all desires are vulnerable!—when you aren't sure whether you can trust someone else to take them, and you, seriously and treat you kindly and respectfully. Remind yourself that trust is a two-way street. Yes, it is partly up to you to choose partners who seem trustworthy and to behave in trustworthy ways where they are concerned. But each of us has that responsibility to the person or people we've chosen to be with. You are not the only person in the relationship who has a responsibility to treat the other right! (One of the things you might want to add to your "things I want in a relationship" list is "someone of proven trustworthiness.")

Your desires, wants, and needs are just as legitimate as anyone else's. The fact that you are fat, or that you desire fat partners, doesn't mean that your desires are in any way unreasonable or something you should give up on because you don't want to seem too demanding.

On Being a Sex Object

If you were to go solely on the impressions given by mainstream media, you would think that being sexually objectified was one of the most sublime delights available to humankind. Clothes, diets, shoes, makeup, hair products, cars, music, jewelry, household appliances, and much, much more is sold on the promise that these things will render you magnetically attractive and make every man and woman within twenty miles stop and gaze at you in a sort of awed lust. Our whole society is constantly atwitter about what is and isn't sexy, what is and isn't desirable, what's "hot or not."

Some people do indeed enjoy being sexually objectified. For some people it is very affirming to have their desirability reflected back at them in that way. It can be empowering and encouraging to know that your body is such a source of fascination and desire for another person. Some people also get a lot out of having someone react so strongly to their mere presence, and they find it gratifying when they don't really have to do anything special to get a strong reaction.

"I have had partners who couldn't get enough of my hips and there have been others who loved everything that my fat body offered. My reaction to such unabashed fat admiration used to be disbelief, but time, and a steady succession of really fat-lusting lovers, has taught me to not accept anything less than a partner who adores all of my squishiness."

Other people don't enjoy being sexually objectified all that much, or at least not in all circumstances. Being sexually objectified can put one in a bit of a strange place. Objectification is one sided, for one thing: it's all about the objectifier's thoughts and reactions, and it happens whether or not the person being objectified likes it or likes the person doing it. Objectification may not include the whole person, with personality and independence and thought and emotion, but may merely be about some particular physical aspect(s) of that person. For some people, being sexually objectified can feel a little bit like having someone talk about you as if you weren't in the room.

For some people, and fat people particularly, being sexually objectified can also bring up reactions that include fear, self-doubt, and suspicion. The culture we live in tells us, repeatedly and for years on end, that our fat bodies are not worthy of being desired, that it is basically impossible for us to be objectified in any sexually positive way. We may learn to hate our own bodies and be able to think of them only in negative terms, and we may even think of specific body parts (bellies often come in for particular loathing) as being unacceptable under any circumstances.

Especially if you have learned to feel this way about your body, having someone else objectify it or lust after it can be profoundly unsettling and disturbing. It may take you by surprise, it may shock you, and it may make you enormously uncomfortable and self-conscious. Even if you have a good body image, being objectified can still feel weird. If you have not had a lot of experiences with being objectified (or at least not ones you knew about!), you may not know what to think of it or what to do about it.

Fortunately, you don't actually have to do anything about it. Objectification is not something for which you have to assume any responsibility. It is completely and totally about the person doing the objectifying. You do not have to feel grateful for being objectified. You don't have to feel aroused or pleased by it unless you actually are. And even if you do like it (which you might!),

"The first time I was with a man who was attracted just because I'm a big woman, I was so turned on by it that the sex was amazing!"

you certainly don't have to put out sexually just because someone else objectifies you. You don't owe anyone anything just because they take an interest in you or your body. Their interest is *theirs*.

So what do you do about being objectified? The real question is: what do you want to do about it? Do you want it to just stop and go away? You can tell the person to cut it out, or you can remove yourself from the situation. Do you want to simply pay no attention to it and carry on with whatever you were doing? You can do that, too. You can use it as an opportunity to start a conversation or to deepen one you were already having. If you think you might be as interested in the person objectifying you as that person seems to be in you, you can flirt. You can offer the person your phone number. Or you can just wait and see. Whether or not someone objectifies you is not really up to you: you can't really stop that person from doing it except by removing yourself from the situation. What *is* up to you is whether you want to do anything about it.

Sometimes it's hard to believe in other people's attraction to us. It's not only fat people who have this problem, as anyone who has ever read more than a couple of fashion magazines can tell you. Our society encourages people, and especially women, to believe that their bodies are never good enough, never attractive enough—that even the tiniest flaw is enough to make other people run for the nearest air sickness bag.

This is not, in fact, true. We know this. But try telling that to the part of your hindbrain that has been trained your whole life to believe that only bodies that are perfect in every way are truly worthy of desire and lust and love.

"A few times I've been approached by so-called 'chubby chasers,' and those experiences always left me feeling extremely uncomfortable, borderline unsafe. For those men, it seemed like their attraction was less about wanting my fat body and more about wanting to have sex with someone they thought wouldn't say no."

So what should you do when someone tells you that you're desirable, that you're pretty or cute or lovely or sexy or handsome or drool-worthy or fuckable or what-have-you? Regardless of whether or not you are interested in following up on it, or having anything to do with the person in question, you still have to process the knowledge and make sense of the experience. How do you stop yourself from dismissing it out of hand, assuming that it can't really be true, or telling yourself that the person doesn't know what she's talking about?

There are several things you can do. First, you can assess whether the expression of interest seems genuine and respectful or not. People can express desire kindly and charmingly, and they can do it rudely and crassly. They can even do it insultingly. If you don't like the way someone is expressing interest in you, you can simply disregard it. Or you can, if you like, say, "Stop being a jerk!"

For those expressions of interest that do seem genuine, kind, and okay, on the other hand, you can begin simply by giving that person the benefit of the doubt. It doesn't matter if you agree with the person that you are hot or cute or handsome or what-have-you. Attractiveness is not a matter of fact; it is a matter of opinion. Other people are entitled to an opinion, whether or not you happen to agree with it. People give compliments and express attraction and desire as praise and tribute, and to have those compliments and expressions refused is basically like telling someone that those feelings don't count or aren't valid. That's probably not what you intend to communicate when you refuse to take a well-meant, kindly phrased compliment, but that is, in effect, what you are saying, and it's ungracious and rude and it shuts the other person out.

Second, you can say "thank you" to a compliment. Many of us, male and female, fat and thin, have been socialized to deflect compliments and praise, to say things like "Oh, it was nothing" or "Don't mention it" or "That's very nice of you to say," which is particularly insidious, because it attributes the compliment to the other person's kindness rather than assuming it's genuinely how they think or feel. We will redirect praise and expressions of interest onto our clothes, our makeup, even the lighting in the room. Many of us are also very good at changing the subject. It can be a real challenge to just say "Thank you" and let the compliment or comment stand. This is exactly why it's worth doing.

"Many of my 300+ sexual partners were interested in me because of my fat. When I was a teenager I didn't quite understand it so much, but as I grew older (and explored pansexuality) I discovered that my fat was a powerful attraction in and of itself for more than a few men."

Third, you can consider accepting someone else's expressions of interest as an exercise in trust. Trusting people to be kind and not cruel, when it comes to your physical self, can be very hard. It is difficult for good, sensible reasons. But when the person who is expressing their attraction or desire is someone you already trust in a sexual sense—or is someone you would like to trust in that way—then it is especially important to be able to trust that person when she or he tells you something.

Finally, you can file declarations of attraction and desire away in some little drawer of your memory, and, later on, take them out and try seeing yourself through the eyes of the person who paid you the compliment. Having someone tell you that you have pretty eyes or great skin or sexy shoulders might make you look at your reflection a little differently. Having someone tell you how sexy you are and how much they'd like to show you a good time might make you think a little more of your sex appeal. In private, and without the pressure of

continued on page 91

What is it like for you when a partner reacts positively to an aspect or part of your body about which you yourself aren't so positive?

"My current partner is very verbally and physically positive toward my belly, which I had previously been very self-conscious about and had dealt with negativity from partners in the past because of it (the belly size, not my self-consciousness—that's a whole separate issue). It has been very healing for me to be with someone who really likes my belly."

"I remember when my ex-fiancée said that she liked the overall 'thickness' of my body. That was hard for me to take in at the time. My wife has also made positive comments about my breasts, a part of my body I have a really hard time liking. I tend to be really mean about my breasts, despite my knowing that body hatred is more or less like internalized homophobia—bullshit I've consumed from the larger culture."

"Every partner who's reacted positively to any aspect of my body below the neck (aside from my hands, which I rather like independent of outside feedback) has inspired doubt and some distrust in me, because I feel negatively (or neutrally at best and after many years of work) about most of my own body. Not so much when it's clothed and functioning—but when it's being looked at or touched by someone else? Brrrr, scary."

"My upper arms are huge, they are considerably larger than my forearms, and they've always been the least favorite part of my body. I hated them for years, never wore sleeveless tops, and was ashamed of the fact that I don't really have elbows, just fat. My boyfriend really likes them, and for the most part I think it is strange. I mean, he will do things like tell me he loves my arms and thinks they are sexy, which definitely makes me feel better about them. I recently took to wearing sleeveless tops for the first time in my life. I don't think that he's the only reason I've decided to let go of my issues, but he has played a part in it."

"For a long time I was very self-conscious about how big my thighs are. One day I sent a photo of myself from the waist down reclining on my bed in a pair of sexy panties to a guy I had been talking to, and he mentioned that he loved my 'thick thighs.' Since then I've had many others comment on them. These comments have helped me to feel less self-conscious about a part of my body that I had previously been somewhat disgusted with. Now, I love my thighs. Of course, this is not purely due to positive reinforcement coming from outside sources— I've definitely made a lot of progress as far as the way I feel about myself goes."

"I always avoided my belly, and most partners would kind of skim over it. But my husband will grab a handful and growl at me, which I like."

"My primary partner loves my soft belly, and even after nine years, it's a little difficult for me to believe she's sincere. She likes to kiss and play with my squishy belly fat. I have names for the two parts of my body that I feel most negatively about, my overhanging belly (my 'apron,' ugh, terrible word) is Muffin and my double chin is my Agnes. She was touching me lovingly on both occasions when those bits became named. Her sweet affection really helped me own Muffin and Agnes and have more love toward them. These are still the parts I'm most self-conscious about, but they are mine now, and in private I don't hate on them anymore."

continued

"I had a lover once who insisted on undressing me and not allowing me to hide myself. It was a new and terrifying experience for me. He spent a lot of time in the undressing process and he seemed almost like he was inspecting me, but the only comments he made while doing so were comments of praise. He seemed to focus those comments primarily on the parts of me that he could sense I was uncomfortable with (my belly, thighs, etc.). When he was done, he pushed me backwards onto the bed and got up over me on all fours and said, 'You must come to understand here (as he placed his hand over my heart) and not just here (as he placed his index finger on my forehead) that there is no part of you that is unlovely, unsexy, unacceptable, or unavailable to me at any time. Because if you believe that any part of you is unlovely, unsexy, unacceptable, or unavailable, you will withhold that part of yourself from me, and if I cannot have all of you, I don't want any of you.' It was probably one of the most defining moments of my entire life. No one had ever put it that way before. It did not make an 'instant transformation' in me, but I went home that night and stood in front of the mirror naked and really looked at me and started asking the question 'what is "wrong" with what I am seeing and who gets to decide what constitutes "right" or "beautiful" from "wrong" or "ugly"?' I kept that practice up until I could look at me and not make judgments and from that carried those feelings over into how I saw others. It was very liberating and finally allowed me to see myself as beautiful, vibrant, and sexy."

having to respond, it is a little easier to explore the potential and the positive aspects of other people's interest and attraction. If you take a little time to think about the fact that people may indeed consider you a sex object, you'll likely feel less blindsided when it happens. That makes it easier to deal confidently and pleasantly with compliments and expressions of attraction and desire as they happen.

The Naked Truth

There's no doubt about it: taking off your clothes means taking off your armor. Clothes are literal armor, protecting us from sun and wind and rain and cold drafts and all manner of scrapes and bumps and insalubrious substances, putting a layer between our skin and anything or anyone that tries to touch us. They act as psychological armor, too, of course. It isn't just the physical protection clothes offer that matters, it's also the control they give us over what is seen and unseen, as well as what kinds of social messages our presence sends. Clothes are also a buffer, a space maintainer that preserves a critical distance between private and public, between our vulnerable individual bodies and other people's ability to see them.

No wonder getting naked makes so many people so nervous. Virtually the only time that we get naked in front of other people—and where those other people have social permission to enjoy a good long look—is when we are with a lover. Especially if the lover is new, this can be very stressful. People of all sizes and shapes get pretty frantic about the prospect of getting naked with someone new. Almost all of us, it seems, have learned to worry that the sight of our naked bodies might be enough to send another person, no matter how sexually interested they seem to be, running for the hills.

For fat people, this fear can be especially intense. The general cultural loathing of fat bodies makes many of us suspicious of even the most enthusiastically expressed desire. We also realize, perhaps more than some thinner people, just how much clothes can be used as a protective mask, and just how big the difference can be between the clothed body and the naked body. All bodies, no matter their size or weight, have their odd lumps and bumps, strange proportions, and saggy or flabby or funny-looking bits, about which we are often exquisitely sensitive. (The fact that we tend not to see these flaws in media depictions of bodies owes a great deal more to editing and Photoshop than it does to the bodies in question.) With fat bodies, though, these various features are often more pronounced: one of the enduring truths about fat bodies is that differences between bodies tend to be bigger because the bodies themselves are bigger. There is, in other words, simply more to see when the clothes come off, and that includes all the various aspects of our bodies that make us nervous or self-conscious.

As uncomfortable as this can be, it's also pretty normal. Most of us would rather feel positive and empowered when it came to getting naked in front of others, a difficult but worthwhile goal. If you don't happen to be there yet, don't kick yourself. Take a deep breath and remember that you're not alone and that most people, even the "beautiful" people, also worry about what other folks think of them when they get naked.

One thing to keep in mind about getting naked in front of a sex partner is that this other person is not in the room to play judge and jury. That person is there out of emotions like excitement, affection, love, lust, and desire. That person is automatically disposed to look at you favorably, and not with the hypercritical, excruciatingly focused viewpoint that many of us use when we look at ourselves. The person you're getting naked for is eager and excited to see what is under your clothes, and, more to the point, to do all the other things that go along with nakedness: feeling, caressing, licking, nibbling, and so on. If you've gotten to the clothes-removal part of the evening, it is highly unlikely that the person you're getting naked for is looking for an excuse to leave.

It's easy to forget, but the person you're with probably has body anxieties to cope with as well. When we're attracted to someone, we tend to see them as being exactly that—attractive. Attractive people don't have to worry about what other people think of them when they take their clothes off, right? Even while we obsess about our own appearance and what our partner(s) are going to think of our nakedness, we tend to hold our lovers to a completely different standard. And they, for their part, are most likely doing the exact same thing with regard to their own bodies and ours.

What it all comes down to, if I may be strictly pragmatic here for a moment, is that you only have the body you have. If you're getting undressed with someone because naked sexy fun time is in the offing, chances are good that your partner has already figured out that you're fat. If your partner has seen and touched you, embraced you, felt you up a bit, and so on, then that person should have a reasonable idea of what's going on under the clothes. It's not as if people's bodies magically transform from thin to fat (or vice versa) just because they take off some garments.

Occasionally, though, there are still bumps in the road. Sometimes, especially for people who are at the thinner end of the fat spectrum or whose bodies conform particularly well to a particular gender ideal—an hourglass figure on a woman, for instance—partners may have an unrealistic idea of what the body under the clothes will look like. Sometimes we wear foundation garments that create a different silhouette or that suggest that gravity has no effect on our plushness. When these come off, there is a different reality for our partners to negotiate. Even art and cartoon images of fat people can leave people with unrealistic ideas of what fat bodies are really like: we are not, as a rule, helium buoyant and perfectly perky in every way!

continued on page 98

INTERVIEW:
Taking It Off for the Camera with Substantia Jones

Substantia Jones is the photographic mastermind behind the size-acceptance photoblog Adipositivity.com. As a fat woman who understands what being looked at and being seen while naked is all about—from both sides of the camera—she shares her insights about nakedness, gaze, and the all-important ingredient of attitude.

Q: *What seem to be the biggest hurdles people face in getting naked for the camera? Do you think that these are similar to, or different from, the kinds of hurdles people face in getting naked in front of a partner?*

A: The biggest hurdles? Our parents. The messages we receive from our parents during the formative years, which inform our body image. These messages are too often shame based. We then go on to absorb the lessons taught us by media and popular culture, most of which are fueled by economic greed and judgmentalism. Religion, the weight loss industry, corporate medicine, mainstream fashion. Unenlightened parents get lots of help. And yes, all this can affect our comfort in getting naked for any reason, including for a partner.

I've been known to clutch my pearls when told of some of the negative body messages people have heard from their parents. But upon reflection, I often realize I heard the same things, sometimes word for word, from my own parents. But after years of drinking the Kool-Aid (to wash down the diet pills), I've come to embrace a healthier relationship with my fat body.

Q: *What do you enjoy about photographing fat nudes?*

A: Being a fat woman, I have a personal stake in adjusting how fat folk are regarded, aesthetically and otherwise. I also have a strong empirical belief that it's possible to do so through bombardment of visuals.

And there's usually a lot of laughing that goes on during shoots. There has to be. You're getting naked for a stranger with a camera and a somewhat unusual notion in mind. So yes, loads of laughs, and quite a bit of fuck-you-ism at the thought of hate-filled sizeists looking at our fat, dimpled asses. We are comrades in the fight. In our birthday suits.

Q: *What makes nakedness sexy? Or unsexy? (Does the answer change depending on whether you're in photographer mode? If so, how?)*

A: I think for most of us, whether or not a naked body is sexy depends largely on context. When I'm making photographs, I make an effort to avoid certain of the trappings of "sexy." Nevertheless, that's exactly how many describe the resulting images. And I get that. You're looking at a woman who, because of her size, society has insisted remain largely hidden. Yet she's uncovering her body for you, in a dominant, contrarian, almost outlaw manner. That combination of intimacy and power can be fiercely hot.

Q: *What advice would you give to someone who wanted to learn to be more comfortable getting naked in front of another person?*

A: Practice, practice, practice! Mystery breeds fear. Relieve some of the mystery by being naked with yourself (and your mirror) as often as is practical. Make sure you've laid eyes on every inch of you, at least once. Squatting over a mirror is not just for tick season!

continued

And those who'd tell you anyone who prefers a big partner is a freak? Fuck 'em. One who appreciates your fat body, the way it is today, is no more fiendish or odd than one with a preference for blondes. Choose a partner who'll revel in every part of your "you-ness," including your physical being, adoring every wobbly bit of it. Hungrily. And when they tell you you're beautiful, believe them.

Q: *In your experience, how does photography affect people's comfort with their own nakedness?*

A: Sadly, photography is far more often used as a tool for inducing body shame than it is as a confidence builder. (There's more money in the former than the latter.) But it can obviously be used to promote happiness and pleasure, as well.

For folks already fighting a belief that they're inferior because they're fat, it's just a short jump to feeling inferior because they're shaped a certain way, or not shaped another. I've had fat women who visit my website regularly tell me they held their breath until they saw an Adipositivity image that resembled their own body. (The wait can sometimes be long, as fat bodies are abundant not only in volume, but in variety. I've seen more naked fat women than a Lane Bryant fitting room, and I've never seen two alike.) I think this speaks to the fact that we all want to see ourselves represented in media. Even neutral depictions of marginalized groups can make valuable contributions toward our sense of belonging.

Q: *In your experience, how does attitude affect the way people look when they're naked?*

A: I love this question! And *attitude* is often the word I use to elicit a bolder response from a subject. I'll sometimes give a direction like

"Give me exuberance" or "Give me superhero." But more often, I'll ask an Adiposer to "give me 'tude." Rather than telling them how to feel for the camera, I'm requesting that they simply reveal how they feel for the camera. The same naked body can repel us, then attract us a moment later, the only change being the disposition of the embodied. One of many things the right attitude can do for you.

Q: *If you could tell every fat person three things about nakedness, what would you say?*

A: Focus on the functions your body can perform for you. Does your body provide you pleasure? Locomotion? A means of communication? A host for adornment? A pillowy seat? Embrace your vessel Adore it for its accomplishments. Work what works.

Go skinny-dipping! I lived far too many years without doing this, but now that I have, I desire this unrivaled pleasure daily. Until you've chunky-dunked, it's difficult to grasp how even a few tiny inches of swimsuit can block the sensation of moving water lapping and massaging you, drawing your attention to the normally tucked-away bits of your body that have never before felt this sort of delight. Get naked and get wet.

Don't hide. Masking your perceived "flaws" only calls attention to them, saying to people, "I'm negatively conscious of this part of me. You should be, too." Unhappy with a body part? Tattoo it. Reveal it. Wrap it in bold patterns. Let it shake, jiggle, and swing. Decide what role that part has in making/keeping you happy and healthy, then allow it to do so, without hindrance.

So it is true that sometimes people will be genuinely surprised by the reality of a naked fat body. Sometimes the reaction will be graceful and gracious, and sometimes it won't. The responsibility to be gracious, however, is theirs. If you are taking the leap of trust required to get naked in front of someone else, the least that person can do is be courteous.

As I said before, you only have the body that you have, at any given moment in time. That's all anyone has. Luckily, that's enough, and the body you have is capable of giving and receiving wonderful pleasure, even if you get a little worried about whether other people are going to like it. Assuming that your partner will not appreciate your body is just borrowing trouble. Assuming that your partner will take pleasure in your body, on the other hand, creates an environment in which that is expected and welcome. You don't have to be a Pollyanna about it, but neither do you need to shut out the possibility of a very pleasant surprise.

The Belly Dance

The thing about bellies, as I have told many people over the past decade, is that they're what lie between our hearts and our genitals. Literally and figuratively, they are in the middle of everything that we do that is in the remotest way physical, and that absolutely includes our sex lives. Of all the places that human bodies carry fat, the belly is the one with which people seem to struggle the most.

The fat belly is symbolic of the fat person, of fatness itself. "Belly and butt" shots festoon nearly every mainstream media news report on fatness. "Belly fat" is blamed for everything from cancer to constipation. Flat stomachs and six-pack abdominal muscles have come to be the tabloid standard of what a "good body" is to such an extent that whenever a woman celebrity appears in public with any visible roundness to her abdomen whatsoever, celeb-watchers immediately snap to attention, speculating about whether the celeb in question is now sporting a "baby bump" or is merely "getting fat." Even a normal rounded belly on a lean person is likely to be looked at with derision or at least suspicion. A belly that is actually fat is beyond the pale.

Bellies are also used as a focus of specifically sexual humiliation. Hanging belly "aprons" on women that overlap or include the mons are often cruelly mocked as "gunts" (gut/cunt) or FUPAs (Fat Upper Pubic Areas). Fat men are derided for having such big bellies they can't see their penises when they look down. Women of all sizes get so worried about their bellies, and about the possibility of others disapproving of them, that they may find it next to impossible to wear a swimsuit or get naked in front of others, let their lovers touch their bellies or abdomens, or enjoy sex. It's altogether too easy to view your belly as the enemy, as the physical manifestation of everything that is infuriating, embarrassing, or painful about being fat. The fear and loathing so many of us feel toward our bellies, and the harm this does to our ability to enjoy our bodies, our sexuality, and our lives, attest to the power of the fat hatred that saturates our society.

Bellies can provoke an enormous amount of emotion. Perhaps this is partly because they're where we feel a lot of emotion: we talk about "gut feelings" and "butterflies in the stomach" and "belly laughs" and things that "turn the stomach." There is a sense that the belly is the core of who we are, unmediated, reactive, and real. When we learn to despise our bellies, we are, in that same sense, hating that aspect of ourselves and refusing to trust it. Having another person show kindness to your fat belly, let alone find it erotic, can present a powerful emotional and psychological challenge.

On the other hand, bellies can also be the conduit for a lot of pleasure. Reclaiming your belly from the generalized haze of belly hate and belly fear can be a powerful thing. You needn't be a belly evangelist, although some people certainly come to feel that way. Even if all you ever manage is to look at and touch your body without judging it, just accepting it as part of yourself, you will have done something that many people are never able to do regardless of their weight or size.

When you are not mentally alienated from your belly, it can do wonders for your sex life. Being open to the sensations that happen in your belly, from the butterflies in your stomach to the sway and jostle of belly fat, can produce a sense of being centered and grounded as well as simply feeling good. When you aren't thinking about how your belly looks, or trying to hold it in or control it or stop it from jiggling, you will breathe more freely and more deeply, and you may find that your hips move more easily and with more range of motion too.

Many global traditions that recognize the ways energy moves through the body, including traditional Chinese medicine, Tantra, and several martial arts traditions, identify a pathway that connects the head, the heart, the belly, and the genitals. Without the belly, the head and the heart would have a hard time linking up with the sexual organs. Even if you don't buy in to these theories, the physical fact that the belly is the literal center of the body does seem to lend some credence to the idea that it is also part of a full-bodied experience of sex.

So how do you learn to love your belly, or even tolerate it? There are many paths, and many things that people do, for themselves and for those they love, that help. Simply making a conscious effort not to repeat negative statements or engage in negative thinking about your belly is a great place to start. Touching and massaging your belly, or letting someone else do it, in a way that feels nice to you is another way to get more comfortable with its presence and substance. Try looking at it as if you were looking at a piece of sculpture, paying attention to the swells and rises and dips and valleys, and see if you can't begin to see it as something that

"My partner loves my bellies and has even named both of them—'Esteban' and 'Pouchy.' I love that she chose a word ('Pouchy') that could have negative connotations, but she uses it lovingly and affirmatively. I've been self-conscious about my belly, but her love for it helps. I also have a super pear shape, and my partner is very supportive of my body in a way I'm not always able to be."

is visually interesting in its particular combination of shapes. Deep breathing exercises can help, particularly if you use your stomach and abdominal muscles to help make the breath as long and deep and slow as you can. Some people like to get creative with their bellies. Pregnant women sometimes have belly-painting parties to celebrate the impending birth of a child. Why not get a friend and some makeup and face paint and decorate each other's bellies? Silly fun can be an excellent way to detoxify your relationship with your belly. Another creative option is belly dance. Many belly dancers of a variety of sizes credit dancing with making it possible for them to embrace their bellies. Whatever you can dream up that you think might work for you is worth trying.

> "After years of self-hatred, I ended up tattooing JOY on my belly to help me start celebrating ALL of my body."

Friendly Fire

Friends and family have an unerring knack for pushing one's buttons. This, of course, is because they helped install them in the first place. No one can get under your skin quite as effectively or quite as easily, and no one's nastiness is harder to rise above or keep in perspective. It's hard not to take even the most rote expressions of anti-fat prejudice personally when they come from friends and family, because, after all, you have a personal relationship with those people. Because of all this, it can be exceptionally difficult to cope with whatever nastiness your family or friends may bring your way when it comes to your body, your self-image, your sexuality, your desirability, or your relationships.

> "My family loves me but harasses me every goddamn day of my life about my weight. My family thinks I sleep with women because I can't get a man, and then I get a man and they think I can do better if I were not fat. It's ridiculous."

How you deal with this will depend a great deal on your specific family and friends and how they are likely to react to you pushing back. Some family dynamics are more changeable than others, some individual people are better able to change their ways than others, and some people are more willing than others to acknowledge when they've done wrong by someone and to try to make amends. There is, therefore, no advice that will work in every case or for every person.

> "My mom chastised a friend who was fat-hating on a man she was dating. The woman said something about how would she even have sex with him. You know, that whole trope. Quite offended, my mom told her, 'My daughter is fat and her boyfriend is fat and they have a great sex life!' My mom got the honorary fat acceptance advocate award that day."

The one person whose actions and reactions you do have some control over is you. You can choose how, or even whether, you want to respond to friends and family who do things like put down your appearance, say you won't find a partner, or make you the butt of "jokes" about fat people and how undesirable and ugly they are. You may also be able to choose whether that kind of behavior is something you are willing to expose yourself to. Getting up and leaving the room, or even the house, is not an option in absolutely every case, but often it is, and it certainly gets your point across.

But this may not be necessary. Some people are willing to listen if you stop them and explain that what they are saying is hurtful, even if they thought they were "just playing around." Explaining, firmly and calmly, that what they say isn't true and doesn't reflect the real world can be a very productive wake-up call. Being able to say things like "You know, Uncle Fred, when you say things like that, all I can think is that you must not realize that there a hundred million fat people living in the United States right now, and you're way off base if you think none of us is getting any action" is useful: it makes people stop and think. Being even more direct ("Mom, I know you know I am a fat person. It insults me when you talk about fat people that way; I know you don't think you're talking about me when you talk that way, but I'm fat: you *are* talking about me") can be effective, too. Sometimes people don't think about how what they say sounds to the people around them.

Some people are able to create a détente with family or friends who are hurtful and negative. Other people aren't. It really depends on whether your family and friends are willing to be open to changing their minds and their approaches. Many times, they are. But some people will cling to their prejudices about fat people. This is not your fault. You cannot change it just by trying harder. If someone is unwilling to hear and understand that her behavior is hurting you, no matter how you have tried to explain this, then that person is the problem, not you.

> "At first I think they were a bit scandalized by my approach to fat and sex and so on (I come from a family of mostly women), but then I think it made them feel a little bit empowered themselves. If I, as the fattest person in our family, could find love and sex and be happy, then maybe they could too."

There is nothing you can do that will force anyone to be kinder or more understanding. However, if you are hitting a lot of dead ends with your family or friends over these issues but aren't ready to give up on them, it might be worth seeking out a size-positive therapist or counselor to help you in your dialogue with your family member(s) or friend. Having a third party present who is not invested in preexisting dynamics and relationships can be very helpful.

Strategies and Comebacks

Whenever the legendary burlesque comedienne Belle Barth found herself with a heckler in the audience, she'd give the heckler a frosty glare over the microphone and snarl, "Shut your hole, mine's makin' money." It worked like a charm. For fat people in daily life, dealing with the comments and rudeness of real-life hecklers is not always so easy. But you don't have to get caught without any resources at your disposal. In life as on stage, a little rehearsal and planning ahead go a long way.

continued on page 108

INTERVIEW:
Sheila Addison, Psychologist

Sheila Addison, PhD, is a psychologist with a specialty in marriage and family therapy. She is also a staunch size-acceptance activist. With compassion, insight, and a solid sense of self-protection, Dr. Addison addresses the sticky problem of dealing with family and friends on the issues of sex, love, and fat.

Q: *What to do about parents who are convinced their children won't find love or get married unless said children lose weight?*

A: As a family therapist, I really believe that parents generally want good things for their children and want to protect them from harmful or painful experiences. I think for the most part, parents are not monsters. It is terribly, terribly hard for parents to hear that their well-intentioned actions are, in fact, making things worse. What a devastating thing to have to acknowledge.

I start out with that, because I know firsthand how hurtful it can be to have your parents criticize and pressure you about your weight. But the only way I know for adult children to start to shift their relationship with their parents is to try to understand their parents' perspective just a little bit, as a way of opening the door. Where I'm heading with this is not "learn to see things like they see them, and adopt their view of the world." More like "try on their shoes for a little bit, and see if that stirs up some compassion inside you."

The family therapist Ken Hardy talks about what he calls the VCR model for having "difficult dialogues"—Validate, Challenge, Request. It takes a lot of validation before people are ready for you to challenge them. I think it is possible for these parent/child relationships to change. Family therapy is a great tool if it's available to you, but I haven't lived near my parents since my early twenties, so we've reworked our relationships mostly on our own. It's not easy but it can happen.

Q: *Is there any good way to stop anti-fat talk and fat bashing when it's used as a mode of social bonding among friends or acquaintances? What if you not only don't want to play that game but want other people to stop playing it in front of you, and you don't want to lose your friends?*

A: I wish I had a surefire answer for this one, but it still trips me up sometimes. In the workplace, I will often just change the subject to work, because it's hard to fault someone for wanting to talk about work while at work. Levity sometimes works too—I've walked in on those endless good food/bad food conversations over whatever happens to be out for public consumption, and said something like "Eat the cake; don't eat the cake. It's not rescuing kittens from a burning building! If that's the biggest moral dilemma you have today, you're probably having a pretty good day, you know?" I think it takes practice. There is no script that is a foolproof.

Q: *What can a fat person do about parents or other family members who deliberately try to sabotage or undermine the fat family member's attempts to date and have relationships?*

A: An answer to this would be dependent both on the sabotaging behavior and also on the living circumstances of the parties involved. The very general answer is "Set boundaries." Boundaries might be

continued

"My partner and I will be cutting back our Sunday dinner visits to once a month for the time being; my decision is not up for discussion." They might be "I am over eighteen and am old enough to pay for my own phone line/mobile phone; from now on, all my calls will go there." Or they might be "I am moving out of the house and in with a roommate because I think it's time to have space that is just mine."

One might set a boundary by agreeing with one's partner, "We will go for Sunday dinner, but if my family makes you uncomfortable, you squeeze my hand twice and I'll suddenly remember that I've left the stove on." Or by saying "Mom, Grandma, I am bringing a date to Sunday dinner, but I must insist that we find something to talk about other than my weight and President Obama. My date likes orchids and clarinet music, just like both of you, so perhaps we can talk about those things. Otherwise we'll have to cut dinner short."

If you are an adult, you are entitled to a private life and to decide how much of that life you share with your family. You are entitled to take steps to facilitate your privacy and to advocate for yourself and your partner. And your partner is entitled to be informed about the situation and to set hir own boundaries as sie chooses. You and your significant other will fare best if you work as a team. Good luck.

Q: *What are some ways that parents and family members of a fat person could help that person negotiate the slings and arrows of dating and relationships?*

A: Believe that your fat loved one is lovable just as they are. Tell them this, openly and without reservation. Express joy and delight at the wonderful things they bring to your life. If they like themselves just as they are, affirm that this is a fine thing. Set your own preferences and ideals aside. Trust that this wonderful, lovable person will be lovable to others.

Dating is hard for everyone, and "the course of true love never did run smooth." But understand that for fat people, the usual bumps and bruises of dating may be felt more keenly. It's hard not to wonder "Is it because of my size?" when you experience rejection. Hard-won self-acceptance can come tumbling down in the face of a broken heart. In the face of self-doubt, the best thing you can offer is the loving reminder that if someone doesn't appreciate and value you as you are, they are not the right partner for you.

When your loved one has been unlucky in love, it is not the time to start offering "helpful" suggestions about dieting or appearance changes. (When is the right time? I'm inclined to say "never.") If you are smaller in size, realize that offering your own dating/breakup stories in "solidarity" may not be helpful, because you have size privilege your loved one does not, so an attempt to compare your situations may hurt more than it helps.

Being rejected, whether because of your size or for any other reason, can trigger a flood of shame and hurt. Losing a relationship, even a bad one, is often cause for intense grief. Often the best thing you can do is validate, validate, validate. "I know it hurts." "I'm so sorry you're experiencing this." "I wish I could protect you from this because you matter so much to me." "I can see how sad you are." One of the best questions you can ask a person in pain is "How can I be most helpful to you right now?" It's better to ask than to guess, and guess wrong.

I have yet to meet a fat person who has never experienced hateful size-related harassment. For that matter, I have met many people I would've characterized as thin who have experienced it, too. For virtually everyone I know who has experienced size-related harassment, it has had a trickle-down effect, creating problems for their self-image and self-esteem, contributing to feelings of being unattractive, unlovable, and unsexy. Sometimes, fat-related harassment is directly sexual in nature, too, with remarks about how "no one would want you," "too fat to find the hole" jokes, or simply the time-honored phrase "fat and ugly."

For all those reasons, you might as well be prepared to deal with hateful harassment when it comes. It sure beats being taken totally by surprise. It *definitely* beats internalizing such idiotic criticism and letting it influence how you think and feel about yourself, your sexuality, and your love life.

You can take some comfort in the fact that fat harassment is rarely personal. Some sad, benighted, messed-up individuals simply think it fun—and funny—to make other people react. Making other people react, and especially making other people miserable, is their way of feeling powerful.

For these bullies, *fat* is just another rock to throw. Like *fag* and *dyke*, it's a blunt weapon that owes its effectiveness as a weapon to the fact that it taints by association. It works only if it succeeds in making the target feel fearful and ashamed. This is why these kinds of insults work on people regardless of whether they're thin or fat, gay or straight: because it's not necessarily what you are, but what you're afraid of being, that will get you to react.

"When someone makes a rude comment about my weight, I look them in the eye and say 'And? Your point?' Usually they are so shocked that they won't even reply."

What this means is that your best defense is not to be afraid or ashamed by fat—not by being called fat, not by being fat, and certainly not by having someone point out that you're fat. (After all, it's not like you magically become thin as long as no one mentions your size, right?) The reaction on your part that will frustrate fat-bashing bullies the most is not being stung by what they say. Many times it is simplest and easiest not to react at all, to simply rise above the unlovely sewage emitted by your fellow two-legged creatures, and sail on. If you want to, vent about it later with people whom you can trust to be sympathetic. Or just let it roll off your back as the meaningless attention-whoring nastiness that it really is.

Some people have great success in confronting bullies, although you certainly need not trouble yourself unless you're inclined. Using the same principle of not being embarrassed or reactive works well in confrontation, too.

> "I have been known, when people make comments about my size, to go right up to them and say 'I'm sorry, I didn't catch what you said, would you mind repeating that?' They mostly get really red-faced. Once I had one who was a real smartarse and just said it again. So I kept acting like I was hard of hearing and saying 'I'm sorry, I didn't catch that, could you say it louder?' until the guy was practically screaming 'I SAID, DAMN YOU'RE FAT!' in the middle of the shop. Then suddenly he noticed that everyone was staring at him and he stomped off muttering under his breath."

Other times, what you want is to fight fire with fire. In a scene on the recent TV show *Huge*, which depicted teenagers at weight-loss summer camp, Ian, one of the male leads, is taunted with "When you're in the shower and you look down, what can you even see?" Ian replies, "Your mother." Crass, yes, but absolutely spot-on, and a hell of a zinger.

The following are some favorite strategies and comebacks from people who answered the Big Big Love Survey. Use them freely and happily, and remember: don't waste any time taking fat-phobic bullying personally or seriously. After all, the bullies don't.

> "I may be fat, but you are an idiot, and I could lose weight if I wanted to."

> "I'm fat? Why yes, I am. Well spotted, Captain Obvious."

> "The wider the hip, the tighter the grip!"

"I see you've set aside this special time to be an asshole in public."

"I'm fat? Ooo, you must be psychic."

For those out-loud remarks you're not supposed to overhear:

"I'm fat, not deaf. Just thought you should know."

"Yes, I am fat. And you're an asshole."

"You might want to lower your voice; when you speak loudly like that everyone can hear what a jackass you are."

"I'm fat? Is that really the best you can do? Goodness. A hundred thousand sperm, and you were the fastest?"

"I'm not actually fat, but I am very allergic to sizeist bigots. I swell up something awful whenever one is near. There must be one in the room right now."

"The only trouble I have finding dates is making sure they don't all find out about each other, honey."

"Save your breath; you'll need it to blow up your date."

"You know, normally people of your limited intellect and physical appeal attempt to make up for it by having a pleasant personality."

"Why am I so fat? Because every time I fuck your mom, she bakes me a pie."

chapter four

For Fat Admirers Only

People who like, love, lust after, or are just generally fond of fat people—in general or in specific—form a large and diverse group. Yet because our society is so negative about fatness, and so unlikely to admit its charms, many fat admirers spend a long time hiding their interests. This section includes thoughts on being isolated and closeted, coming out, being a good partner and a good ally to fat people, and the FA Four, an ethical guide to being the kind of fat admirer every hottie wants to take home.

Dear Fat Admirer

Welcome! How nice to see you here. I know you may feel a little awkward and self-conscious being here, with your nose in a book about the simultaneously exciting and intimidating subject of fat people and sexuality, but really you don't need to worry about a thing.

First of all, you're not alone. Yes, I realize that you may feel alone. You might feel like the only person in the world who ever ended up falling madly in lust with someone she never expected to—a fat person. Or you might feel like the only person in the world who really likes the "before" pictures in the diet ads a whole lot better than the "after." Think you're the only person who ever wrote erotic Beth Ditto/Gabourey Sidibe fan fiction? The only one who's had wet dreams about the deliciously raunchy things that might happen to you if you were James Gandolfini's pool boy? The only soul in all the world who would like to see the cast of *Huge* in a porno?

Not even kinda. Not even close.

To tell you the truth, you're in excellent company. No one really knows how many of you there are out there in the world, but given that there are about a hundred million fat people in the United States alone, and the vast majority of them are (or will be) in sexual or romantic relationships at some point in their lives, I'd say the odds are that there are also probably millions upon millions of people who like, love, and lust after people of all kinds of different sizes of large. Just like you. Some of them will never admit it. Some of them will never put a name to it. But some of them will admit it and possibly give it a name as well. Maybe they'll even read this book.

You're not all alike, of course. Some of you are male, some of you are female, and some of you are trans folks or intersex. There are plenty of straight guys among you, and those straight men are more likely to use the *fat admirer* phrase to refer to themselves. But there are also straight women who love the chub, as well as gay men, lesbians, bisexuals, and fantastic flirtatious queers of all flavors and predilections.

Some of you are pretty much straight-up vanilla in your bedroom preferences, aside from liking it large and luscious. Others are kinky in some way or another. Many of you are monogamous, some of you are polyamorous, and some of you could go either way, depending on the relationship and the partner. You run the gamut, basically, in all its vast and variable breadth.

What you like specifically in your partners and their bodies varies a lot, too. Some of you only go for the fattest of the fat, some of you only for the people who are barely bigger than average, and many of you go for the many, many people in between. Some of you are equal-opportunity fatophiles. The same goes for what you like to look at. A lot of you groove on big bellies, big butts, big thighs, and big breasts. But some folks dig even more specific things: back fat, a little bit of padding on the instep of the foot, double chins, thick weightlifter necks. And again, some of you don't play favorites—you like it all. There is something for everyone.

Some of you have always loved the looks and the sensations of bigger bodies and have known you were fat admirers from childhood. Some of you just started to realize you've been grooving on fat people or maybe are just coming to admit that you've been doing it for a while now and it isn't going away. Maybe it's taken you years to admit it to yourself that you enjoy fatter bodies. Maybe you've never questioned it. Maybe you're not usually attracted to fat people but have suddenly found yourself totally into one particular fat guy or gal and are trying to make sense of what's going on.

It can sometimes take people years and years to come to terms with the fact that they desire the people and bodies they do. This can be legitimately hard to do when what you desire are things or people that society tells us are undesirable and ugly. It can take a lot of courage and a lot of momentum to be brave enough to say, even just to yourself, that you like what you like and that's okay. Some lucky people get to that point without any major anguish or conflict. Others have a little struggle along the way but get there in the end. Sometimes people wrestle with their fondness for fatness for a very long time.

Wherever you are in your own journey toward accepting yourself and your fat desires is okay. We don't all travel at the same speed. The point is that you dig fat people, and that is absolutely fine. The fact that you dig them in the particular way that you do is fine. You're not alone, you don't have to hide, and you don't have to be ashamed. All you have to do is do your best to be honest, to be caring, to be kind, and to be a good person with regard to fat people and your attractions for them, just like you would if your attractions were completely mainstream.

Welcome to the fat, sexy neighborhood. Enjoy your stay.

Coming Out

When what you desire is something other than what your society tells you is desirable, coming out can be hard to do. It's really tough, for all kinds of good reasons, to be open about the fact that you are attracted to fat partners, or even to an individual fat person. Our society not only proclaims, in a million ways every day, that fat people are ugly, low-class, uneducated, out-of-control slobs; it also implies that only the most perverse of perverts could possibly stoop so low or be so degenerate as to want to have sex with them, or worse still, fall in love with them.

Because of this, people who desire and/or love fat partners face an uphill battle to have their desires and their emotions respected and acknowledged as legitimate. The mainstream that claims that only thinness is desirable is all too ready to declare that fat admirers don't exist, or that if they do, then they are sick, crazy, or fetishists.

Much like LGBTI folks, fat admirers who want their sexuality to be recognized and treated like anyone else's have to go out of their way to articulate and defend their desires and their pleasures. This is difficult in exactly the same proportion that people's reactions to your desires and attractions are negative, judgmental, or hostile.

For quite a few fat admirers, having to deal with the prospect of such harsh reactions is not something with which they've had much experience. This itself can make coming out seem harder and more fraught than it actually is. This is particularly applicable if you're one of the many FAs who can, as they say, "pass for normal." If you yourself are fairly average in size, height, weight, looks, and so on, and especially if you are also heterosexual, you may not have had any significant experience with people being nasty to you because of some aspect of your person or your personality. Either way, you may not think that bringing the judgmental wrath of others down on your own head sounds like a very good deal.

On the other hand, if your desire for fat partners has proven resilient enough that it hasn't gone away despite your being exposed to years and years of society's anti-fat propaganda, chances are good that you are pretty resilient, too. And that's only one of the reasons that I hope that you consider coming out of the fat-admiring closet if you haven't already.

Coming out about your desires and your loves may seem like it will open you up to attack, but actually, it's a pretty good form of self-protection. No one can blackmail you—literally or figuratively—about something you refuse to hide in the first place. People can try to ridicule you, shame you, or make you feel bad about yourself and about your desires, but this doesn't work as well when you've already made the first move and brought the taboo subject out into the open air. When you've already put it out there that you like what you like and that's all there is to it, people quickly get the picture that this is indeed the case and that your sexual interests are not up for negotiation.

The people who are likely to give you a hard time or criticize you because of your attractions or your lovers are much more likely to do so if they think it'll get a rise out of you. Presenting them with a simple statement of fact, ("Actually, I prefer fat partners and always have" or, even more succinctly, "I've never enjoyed a relationship as much as I do my relationship with X") doesn't leave them so much room to argue. If they seem determined to try to fight with you about it anyway, you can calmly inform them that you don't demand that they share your tastes and you will thank them not to demand that you share theirs.

You may still worry about what people will think of you if they know that you love a fat person or prefer fat partners. On one level this is completely understandable. We all worry about whether or not people approve of us, we all worry about what the repercussions might be if they don't, and we all worry about being undermined by a bad reputation. On another level, what other people think is none of your business. No doubt you think uncharitable thoughts about other people all the time; most of us do. Thankfully, most of the time no one else knows about what goes on in our heads, and that's as it should be.

When you do come out, don't be surprised if other people seem not to be shocked. The people who know you well may have already figured it out. Many people have told me, laughingly, about spending months worrying about what they imagined would be tense, fraught coming-out moments with parents and friends, only to have their parents and friends say "Oh, yeah, I knew that. I was worried you were going to tell me you had cancer or something."

As for the possibility of repercussions, well, yes, it exists. Part of the reason that it exists is that there's a lot of unreasoning prejudice and hatred out there when it comes to fat . . . and unconventional desires. Adding your voice to the people standing up and saying "No, I will not accept being treated badly just because of the kind of person I'm attracted to" helps to change the way people think about and treat people with nonmainstream desires—you know, people like you.

continued on page 121

INTERVIEW:
Coming Out with Yohannon

Yohannon is the *nom de guerre* of a well-known FA who has been out, proud, and active for decades in the fat and fat-acceptance communities. For many years he ran the fat sexuality website the Rotunda (www.rotunda.com, now primarily an archival resource), as well as the fat_sex and fat_BDSM mailing lists, which now exist by the same names as communities on LiveJournal.com. As an FA who is both bisexual and polyamorous, Yohannon has had lots of experience with coming out, and he shares it with us.

Q: *What would you say to an FA/chaser who is afraid to come out of the closet?*

A: One of the chief motivations behind books like *Big Big Love* is to give people who still feel like they're the only guy or gal into fat people on the planet that first push into discovering that there are literally millions of fat lovers out there. They just need to be putting the right keywords into the search engines, as it were. The anonymity provided by the Net also gives you the chance to take those first baby steps toward understanding yourself.

If that's not enough, it's cool—you'll come out when you're ready. Just know that it can literally be at any moment, because sometimes you're given an opportunity too good to pass up. Strength in numbers won't guarantee that you won't catch hell from your friends, family, coworkers, and so forth. What it will do is give you the tools to deal with coming out and the possible fallout from admitting that which makes you something other than "normal."

Q: *Have you experienced any negative fallout because of being an out and-proud FA? If so, what happened and what did you do about it?*

A: One of the biggest negatives is that people will accuse me of some-how causing "fatness"—as if my small encouragement for Health at Every Size (HAES) is causing the obesity epidemic itself. Before it was generally accepted that yo-yo and crash dieting caused more weight gain than loss, any attempt to point out that bad diets are bad for human beings got me labeled as someone trying to increase the size of my dating pool. Oddly enough that's the worst of it for me. . . . I've been very fortunate.

Q: *Do you think that the Internet, and the way that a lot of FA activity has moved to the online world, has affected FAs'/chasers' tendencies regarding remaining closeted or coming out? If so, how?*

A: When I first came "out" as an FA, it was 1982. I suspect the school I went to (SUNY Purchase) helped a lot, as there was a very large, very OUT queer contingent on campus, and having a strong sexu-ally diverse community really made space for me to exist. Even then it would be another three years until I began finding the support groups to bolster my confidence in my preference for fat people and then only by blind dumb luck.

Back then NAAFA [National Association for the Advancement of Fat Acceptance] was posting dance event notices in small text ads in the *Village Voice* classifieds—if you didn't know what to look for, a lonely FA would never have known that there was a place for [him or her]. And this was in New York City's gravitational pull! Most of the rest of the country was pretty much a barren wasteland. How does one learn about something if [you] have to know it exists first?

continued

It was always about luck—if you caught the right bit of daytime TV, spotted one of those classifieds, heard word of mouth about those dances, you were halfway there. But then, that first event is HARD. You had no idea what to expect, what the people were like, what the expectations were.

The Net turns all of that around. Now you can inquire in complete anonymity, if you so choose, from any number of online resources. You can see pictures. And never underestimate the power of porn to solidify the sense of what pushes your buttons! So the Net provides a way for FAs to define, explore, and eventually embrace their differences. On the flip side, it also provides people with a means to remain closeted for years, if not their entire lives. I still hear tales from fat people who were developing an online relationship, sometimes even making the segue to real-life encounters, only to discover their exciting new lover is already fully committed to another—skinny—person. Closeted FAs online can use it to get a chance to appease their desire for something outside of their comfort zone with little risk.

Q: *What responsibilities do you think FAs/chasers have—or should have—to provide political and social support to the fat people to whom they are attracted?*

A: Not everyone is, nor should be, political. That is a choice that should be made for the right reasons at the right time. Only the individual can make that decision. That said, I've often noted that just showing love, affection, adoration, and respect to your fat partner in public can be as political an act as picketing the office of a pediatric surgeon who performs gastric bypass on six-year-olds. Holding your sweetie tight and kissing them with obvious attraction can be a revolutionary act.

Risk is part of life. And yes, it is somewhat risky, but it is also a good thing when people stand up for their own human rights and those of others. Your willingness to come out as someone who desires fat people, either in general or just one specific person, makes a statement that our society needs to hear. No one likes being told over and over again that people like them don't exist or that, if they do exist, there's something wrong with them. You do exist. So do lots of other people like you. Some of them are less brave than you and would really benefit from seeing someone like you be out and proud of your desires, not taking any crap. Sometimes people need to see that there are other people like them in the world before they can start feeling okay about the person they are. You can be that person for someone else—it's an enormous gift.

It's also a gift to the people to whom you might very well be attracted. When you're attracted to someone, you often feel conspicuous as hell, like everyone in a ten-mile radius must know. Trust me when I tell you that this is nothing more than your own self-consciousness: other people do not magically know you're into them. You actually have to make clear to them what's going on and that you're not staring at them because they have spinach in their teeth. Remember that a lot of fat people have plenty of experience being stared at for negative reasons. If you come out as a fat admirer, though, fewer people have to wonder whether you're staring because you're thinking "What a shame; she'd be pretty if she weren't so heavy" or because you're thinking "Oh man, what a freaking dream-boat. I wonder if she's single."

Another good thing about coming out is that it's a chance for you to reaffirm a fundamental truth: that there's nothing wrong with desiring and/or loving other human beings. People don't just *want* to be cared for and cared about. They need to be. It's part of what keeps us sane and part of what lets us thrive. These are things that make life better and richer and more interesting. They're also things that bring joy and stress relief and contentment and reassurance and pleasure, things that are part of a good life—and good health—for everyone.

Love, caring, desire, attraction, sex: these are things that absolutely every human benefits from and deserves. And there is absolutely nothing in the world wrong with you for being strong and proud enough to say so.

How Not to Be an Asshole

I'm not gonna pull any punches here, my Fat Admirer friend. Sometimes you folks have it just a little bit too easy.

I know what you're thinking. It's tough out there for a chubby chaser. I get that. But hear me out. Because of the way anti-fat prejudice works, and especially the way that fat people get told day in and day out that no one is going to want them or love them, you do, in point of actual fact, have some things very easy. Not to put too fine a point on it, but you are assured of a lifetime supply of potential partners who most likely have been indoctrinated in the idea that no one will ever think them sexy or lovable or romantically interesting. Many of them have been stuck in a scarcity mentality for years, even decades, believing that they have a snowball's chance in hell of finding someone who would want them. Some are willing to leap at any chance they get, and, no matter how much people like me tell them to keep their standards high and not to compromise too much, are so hungry for love and attention—and so afraid that you might be their only chance—that they'll put up with a lot of crap and overlook a lot of things they oughtn't, just to feel wanted.

This gives you and other fat admirers way more than your fair share of power.

In an ideal world, relationships—no matter how fleeting, regardless of whether they're purely sexual or more romantic or whatever—would be between equals, people who freely choose to be together for mutual pleasure and benefit and who could as easily choose not to without sustaining any serious damage to their quality of life. In the real world, some fat people go through life terrified that no one will ever want them or love them due to their fatness. As a result, that equality is strained and that freedom gets compromised because there seems to be so much at stake, the chances of getting it seem so small, and the threat of being deprived of it once you have it feels so enormous.

As a fat admirer, you are in the position of being able to offer your partners something they really want, something many of them have believed, perhaps for a long long time, they would be unable to have. Your genuine, unfeigned interest in them as fat people and the fact that you actually are attracted to them, bellies and thigh chub and all, is like something out of a dream or a fairy tale, so much so that some of them might not even be able to believe it exists.

As you may already know, the fact that you can offer this, the happy ending, the pot of gold at the end of the rainbow, means that there are a lot of fat people out there who will be more than willing to go out with you, have sex with you, and, indeed, throw themselves at you headlong. People who would be completely out of your league if they weighed fifty or a hundred pounds less will eagerly giggle and flirt with you as if you were the best catch in the world—not because you are the best catch in the world (sorry, truth hurts) but because at their size, they think you're the closest they'll get to having anything at all. The more conventionally attractive you are, the more intense the effect. A good-looking, decently dressed, reasonably intelligent man of "average" weight or size can walk into virtually any BBW/FA or chub/chaser event and have a roomful of hotties all jostling for position to get his attention.

This, I have no doubt, is a damn good time. That kid in a candy store feeling takes a long time to get old, and low-hanging fruit is so easy to pick and so juicy sweet on the tongue. It's fun to feel desirable, to feel competed over, to feel like a prize. It's fun to know you can have—or at least have a better-than-average shot at having—whatever pretty face in the room strikes your fancy. It's fun to have power.

But here's the thing: with great power comes great responsibility, as some wise dude once said. And when you have this kind of power (in this case the ability to pull people's emotional strings like a puppeteer), you have two options:

1. You can man up and learn how to be ethical in your FA-hood.

2. You can be an asshole.

Being ethical is not necessarily easy. It's definitely harder than just standing there being fabulous and taking your pick of the hot chub action. Being ethical means three basic things.

First, you have to know what you really want. For that to happen, you have to be able to be honest with yourself. If what you really want is a lot of hot sex with hot fatties, that's cool, but don't tell yourself—or anyone else—that you're looking for a long-term relationship. Don't even let them think that it might be the case, if it really isn't. And if what you really want is to find someone to marry and raise cocker spaniels with, don't tell yourself that a bunch of one-night stands with people you barely know will help you get there. And don't just go ahead and have those one-night stands, either, if you're only going to discard those partners after the heat of the moment is passed and you remember the whole married-with-dogs plan.

Second, you have to be able to communicate what you want. Now, I know, "communication" is one of those touchy-feely things, and for some of you it may seem a little suspect. I promise, however, that straightforward, honest, responsible, adult communication is actually useful and not wimpy in the slightest. If you can learn how to say what you want and need and feel and think, without getting angry or defensive, or playing stupid passive-aggressive games, you're going to be far ahead of the pack. It will stand you in excellent stead with regard to relationships and in other areas of your life too.

Straightforward, honest, responsible, adult communication means, among other things, having the stones to say, "Hey, I think you're really hot and I want to have all kinds of sweaty sheet-ripping sex with you, but I'm not looking for a relationship right now. Are you down with that?" Or, conversely, "You know, you're really sexy and I am totally flattered, but I think it might be best if we just call it a night. I wouldn't feel right leading you on."

Third, you'll have to actually enforce your boundaries. That means that you put your money where your mouth is. For example, don't say "Thanks but no thanks" but then decide, what the hell, and have sex with the person anyhow. Maybe your boundary is about getting to know someone well enough to find out how experienced they are with polyamory before you date them. Maybe it's figuring out how to gently but firmly insist, "The sex was lovely, thank you, but, like I said earlier, I'm still not interested in spending the entire night in the same bed, so may I call you a taxi?" Whatever the boundary is, knowing it and declaring it and keeping it is what makes you a man or woman of your word.

What you want may be complicated. What you want may change. That's all normal and okay. You may not actually know what you want, and that's okay too, as long as you're clear with the people you date or have sex with that this is the case and they are okay with it. If you want something specific but you don't communicate what you want, it is not other people's responsibility to be psychic and read your mind. If you communicate what you want but you don't enforce boundaries about what you'll accept, it is not other people's responsibility to enforce your boundaries for you.

If you don't articulate what you want and follow through on what you articulate, what you're probably going to end up doing is just taking whatever's available. This is a problem for two major reasons. Taking what's available just because it's there, without communicating about what you want or what your boundaries are, can be misleading to the people who make themselves available. They may very well think that if you take them up on their offer, it means you both want the same things. (Yes, they also have a responsibility to be communicative, clear, and ethical. And maybe they will be. But maybe they won't. Maybe they don't even know how. In which case, it's your job to step up to the plate and show them how it's done.) The other problem with just taking what's available is that it makes it very easy to take advantage of your situation. When you're a fat admirer, that can easily end up meaning taking advantage of other people's willingness, vulnerability, and need.

Your choices regarding how to conduct your relationships, as a fat admirer and as a human being, are up to you. It's about deciding to be what we call, in Yiddish, a *mensch*: a good, self-aware, trust-worthy person.

THE FA FOUR: FOUR ETHICAL PRINCIPLES FOR FAT ADMIRATION

1. Remember that other people are vulnerable, and fat people are sometimes especially so, when it comes to love, attraction, desire, and sex. The keywords here are *gentleness*, *compassion*, and *boundaries*. Pro tip: Having and keeping clear boundaries protects the people you are with just as much as it protects you.

2. You aren't God's special gift to humankind just because you are attracted to fat people. You're attracted to fat people because they're what you like: fatness is what gives you pleasure. Don't pretend you're bestowing some sort of noble kindness on people when really what you're doing is getting your own personal freak on. You're not doing anyone—least of all yourself—a favor by acting like your hard-on is some kind of charity scholarship. It's arrogant, patronizing, and ugly.

3. Don't break your arm patting yourself on the back. It's fantastic if you do all the right things when you're dating a fat partner. When you're thoughtful enough to call ahead about armless

chairs at a restaurant or you rent something bigger than your Mini so that your date will be comfortable when you're driving somewhere together, that's wonderful, and I promise you that it will not go unnoticed or unappreciated. But, for heaven's sake, don't spend the entire evening doing the "Hey, did you notice that I did something especially for your needs?" thing. All it does is call attention to whatever special needs your partner has, undoing the effects of going out of your way to help make them more comfortable.

4. If you wouldn't do it to a thin person, don't do it to a fat person. If you wouldn't lie to a thin person about being already married, don't lie about it to a fat person. If you wouldn't refuse to use a condom with a skinny person, don't refuse to use a condom with a fat one. If you wouldn't go out of your way to avoid being seen in public with a thin partner, what the hell do you think you're doing trying to avoid being seen in public with a fat one? Grow a spine and face the fact that the people you are attracted to are people, and any person to whom you are attracted is a person to whom you owe at least basic human honesty, dignity, and respect.

Axis of Allies

As someone who desires, cares for, and loves fat people, you have a vested interest in their sanity, health, and happiness. Certainly it's unfair for fat people to bear so much cruelty and harassment just because they're fat, and certainly the world would be a better place if everyone, including fat people, got a little more respect. Which is exactly why you, as a person who has a vested interest in the happiness and health of fat people, need to know how to be a good ally to the fat people you love and care about.

Not every fat person needs or wants the same things from an ally; not everyone needs the same things in terms of support. You can, and should, ask the fat folks in your life what would work best for them. This is true even if you're fat yourself and have your own ideas about what kind of support would be helpful. People's needs and opinions vary. In the survey for this book, respondents were asked what kinds of things partners and lovers could do in order to be better allies. The following represent the most common requests.

"Don't be ashamed of me. Go out in public with me. I want to meet your friends. Someday maybe even your mom."

"If someone makes a nasty remark about my size in my presence, it would be nice if the person I was with got my back. I can defend myself and I will. But it would be nice to know that I wouldn't have to do it all myself, that I'd have backup."

"I like it when someone I am dating takes the time to make sure I will be physically comfortable and is willing to be flexible and change plans if things aren't comfortable or accessible for me."

"The best thing for them to do is to let me know how much pleasure they take in my body. Becoming sexually active in my early twenties was actually the first step in my path to discovering fat acceptance. I started to wonder why I had issues with my body, when my lover was so clearly into it."

"A fat-positive sex partner provides an important sense of sensual affirmation that is sacred and special."

"They can speak up against discrimination when they see it. They can understand that I don't always like my body or feel attractive, and be supportive when that happens. They can tell me and show me that they find ME attractive. And they can regard me as the ultimate authority on my body. For instance, I am a fat person. If someone says to me

'You're not fat!' (by which they usually mean 'You're not ugly!') they aren't respecting that I know my body and I am the ultimate authority on it."

"By taking me out in public and being proud of my appearance. By calling friends on their fat phobia, even when I'm not there."

"Take my needs seriously. Remember that I am a (very) grown adult with a good sense of what I need and when I need it and that it means a lot to have helpful but not ego-based support. Remember that I want to help you, too, when you need it. Remember that I have to think about all this way more than I want to. Remember that real help that is really about wanting good things for me will make me want to shag you rotten."

"Oh my gosh, my wife is the BEST ally and advocate. She has helped me get more positive and assertive about what I need. She has called people out on their stuff. She has encouraged me to read particular blogs, to get more involved in HAES [Health at Every Size]-philosophy stuff, all kinds of things. Her utter lack (as far as I can tell) of fat phobia is one of the great blessings in my life."

"It's important for a partner to be on your side—whether that means discouraging fat jokes among peers or openly expressing love for your body. That can take a lot of bravery and certainly a willingness to be misunderstood or discriminated against in turn, but I certainly don't want to waste my time on a coward."

"Don't pester about food or weight issues, EVER. Don't blame people's health issues on their weight, even if the doctor does, because it's NOT YOUR PROBLEM. Remember that health is not morality. That what you eat is not morality. That what you look like is not morality—or any sort of indication of what sort of person your partner is. We do not live in Fairy-Tale Land, where inside beauty always shows up as thinness and blondness—thank goodness."

"My husband is the best supporter when it comes to size/weight discrimination; he shares my belief that fatness is not a negative trait, he expresses his love for my body and my being frequently, and he publicly opposes sizeism and supports individuality. It is very clear to me and to others who know him that he values self-expression and non-judgmentalism in all forms, and to me this is the best support he could possibly give me against size/weight discrimination."

"I think a lot of guys are secretly sexually attracted to fat people. They like having sex with us and spending time with us, but they're embarrassed to have an actual romantic relationship and will save that for a more 'marriageable' or 'high status' or 'thin' partner because they don't want to go against cultural norms or take ribbing from friends and family. I'd like to see a lot of those 'secretly attracted' people give a little more of themselves to their relationships, and I'd like to see us fatties demand a little more in our relationships."

"Hold my hand in public. Seriously. I definitely feel the effect of thin-partner privilege. I hear almost no comments/shaming from strangers when I'm with my husband. It's far more regular than I'd like when I'm alone."

"Listen and understand when I experience frustrations, and file away the information for when it's necessary. My husband is better at remembering which theaters and venues have seats I can sit in vs. ones that are [narrower] than I am, for example."

"Listen to what kind of help or allyship I'm asking for. Stand up for someone being discriminated against. When someone is making stupid comments about weight, speak up and fight against it. Let other thin people know that you are an ally to fats. Let me vent about being treated poorly due to my weight. Come with me to the gym and work out next to me."

"One major way is self-education. Do some reading about Health at Every Size, and about fat phobia. Being able to have an intelligent conversation on the topic without having to do 'Fat 101' every time is important to me. Be willing to work on breaking fat-phobic habits, especially in casual daily speech. It takes time, and it feels weird at first, but it does matter to me."

"I'm a person of color and when people react to my ethnicity and handle it like a precious knickknack, it feels weird. So would someone who felt the need to talk at all about my size and appearance. So the way a sexual/romantic partner can be a supporter is just to see ME, not my race, not my size."

"I believe in the Show-Don't-Tell method: hold my hand, put your arm around my shoulders, smile and keep eye contact, the things any couple does to show that glow. And if someone DOES say 'WTF, why are you with the Fat Chick?' well, then you Tell. Tell them whatever it is that put you at my side, my sparkling wit, my sarcastic humor, my enthusiasm in bed, my oral fixation, my love of action movies and spy novels and playing D&D. Whatever it is, tell them. And then tell them that it really isn't any of their concern, since I'm taken, and so are you."

"Treat me like a normal person. I am a normal person."

chapter five

To Your Health!

It's hard to feel sexy if you don't feel good. And it can be hard to get the kind of caring and competent medical care you need when you're fat. This section gives you tools to negotiate both sets of hurdles involving weight, health, and sex. It also walks you through the sexuality side of some common fat-related health conditions like polycystic ovary syndrome, lymphedema/lipedema, and gynecomastia. Additional tips help you slash your risk of a sexually transmitted infection, injuring yourself or a partner during sex, and becoming pregnant if you don't want to be.

Your Rights as a Fat Sexual/Reproductive Health Care Consumer

1. You have the right to be respected as a sexual being with a bona fide sexual identity and relevant sexual experiences, regardless of your weight or size.

2. You have the right to be treated considerately and competently with regard to any sexual health question, issue, or problem, no matter what your weight or size.

3. You have the right to a conscientious, competent, compassionate, and thorough medical examination in which weight and size come into play only insofar as they are actually medically relevant.

4. You have the right to a health care provider who is aware that fat patients sometimes require special accommodations and/or techniques and who is willing to make reasonable efforts to provide those things where needed.

5. You have the right to be spoken to, touched, handled, and treated with respect and gentleness no matter your size, shape, or weight.

6. You have the right to have your sex, gender, and orientational identities respected by your medical practitioners.

7. You have the right to work with a nonjudgmental medical practitioner who understands that people of all sizes may choose to engage in a wide variety of safe, sane, healthy, consensual sexual activities and participate in a wide variety of relationship patterns.

8. You have the right to have your contraceptive and safer sex needs taken seriously and addressed professionally, regardless of your weight or size.

9. You have the right to obtain treatment, get referrals to specialists, and be prescribed medications, where relevant, without being required to lose weight first.

10. You have the right to sexual/reproductive health care that acknowledges that sexuality is a complex realm of life that may involve many social factors, including size/weight and size/weight discrimination, and that these things may affect health and access to health care.

Fertility, Contraception, and Pregnancy

Ever heard the one about how fat girls can't get pregnant? There's no punch line, because it's not a joke: fat women get pregnant all the time.

There is some research that indicates that fat women and men may be less easily fertile than thinner people for a variety of reasons that range from hormone levels to PCOS (polycystic ovary syndrome; see page 153) to thyroid issues, but the relationship between fatness and fertility is neither particularly clear nor well understood. Research presented by groups including the American Society of Reproductive Medicine suggests that in some cases it may take longer for fat people to conceive. However, there is absolutely no reason to expect that any given fat person is, or will be, infertile.

In general, fat people who are sexually active but who are not trying to conceive have the same need for contraception as anyone else does. In general, fat people can use the same contraceptive methods as anyone else, too.

There are five basic types of contraception.

- Barrier contraceptives work by keeping sperm and eggs from coming into contact. Barrier contraceptives include condoms, diaphragms, Lea's Shield, and cervical caps.

- Intrauterine contraceptives (IUDs, intrauterine devices) are small devices that are inserted into the uterus to prevent a fertilized egg from implanting in the wall of the uterus. Some of them also incorporate timed-release hormones to further enhance their effectiveness.

- Oral contraceptives are a hormonal contraceptive that comes in pill form. They prevent pregnancy by suppressing ovulation and by preventing fertilized eggs (if they are present) from implanting in the uterus.

- Nonpill hormonal contraceptives include skin patches, under-the-skin implants, vaginal inserts, and injections.

- Sterilization is permanent birth control that makes someone infertile. It can be achieved by vasectomy for men or by tubal ligation or the Essure procedure for women.

For more information on birth control methods and how each works, consult your doctor or clinic. For general online information, see PlannedParenthood.org or the Association of Reproductive Health Professionals website at arhp.org.

Contraceptive effectiveness may be a problem for some fat people. About 10 percent of the respondents to the Big Big Love survey—a fairly significant proportion—reported having experienced difficulties with contraception due to weight or size. There is evidence that suggests that fat women using hormonal contraception may experience higher failure rates than thinner women. It is not entirely clear why hormonal contraceptives fail for some fat women while others can use them without any problems. Increased failure rate of hormonal contraceptives in fat women may be due to inadequate dosage, meaning that some fat women might require higher doses of the hormones in question because their bodies are larger. It is also true that fat women are more likely to have underlying hormonal imbalances such as PCOS, which is highly correlated to fatness. Such endocrine disorders can change how effective contraceptives can be. There may be additional factors we don't yet know about. Fat women who use hormonal contraceptives may wish to use a backup contraceptive like an IUD or condoms as well. The effectiveness of diaphragms and cervical caps can also be affected by changes in weight: your doctor can advise you on the fitting protocols for your particular device and let you know what you should look out for to know if it's time to have a refitting.

Pregnancy and fatness are controversial, to say the least. Many medical sources claim that there are significantly higher risks of complications when fat people become pregnant. Risk is not the same thing as inevitability, however. Most fat people's pregnancies proceed in a completely textbook fashion, while some thin people's pregnancies involve complications. If you are pregnant or are planning to become pregnant, discussing it with a fat-friendly obstetrician or midwife is an excellent idea. Assembling a fat-friendly medical team that will be respectful of you, your pregnancy, and your baby-to-be may be challenging. Asking fat friends who are parents about their experiences is one good way to get recommendations for medical professionals with whom you will be able to work happily.

There are numerous things that those who are pregnant or who plan to become pregnant can do to improve their odds of a healthy pregnancy and a healthy baby. Chief among these is to make sure that you consume plenty of folic acid, a nutrient that is necessary for proper nervous system development in the fetus. Because there is evidence that babies born to fat parents have a higher incidence of the kinds of birth defects that can be prevented by adequate folic acid, fat parents-to-be should be especially careful to get enough of this critical nutrient.

Sexually Transmitted Infections and Safer Sex

If you can catch a cold, you can catch a sexually transmitted infection (STI). Fat does not protect anyone against STIs. The microorganisms that cause infections don't know, and don't care, how much you weigh. There is not a virus in the world that only infects people who wear smaller clothing sizes and leaves the fatter folks alone. Just like the flu or food poisoning, STIs are equal opportunity illnesses.

No doubt you already know that STIs are serious business: some of them can kill you. Even the nonfatal ones are a whole bunch of no fun and can cause pain, scarring, infertility, and cancer. Several of them are caused by viruses. HIV, which causes AIDS, is a virus, but human papilloma virus (HPV), hepatitis, and herpes are all viral as well. These cannot be cured. Some others can be cured, but unless they are nipped in the bud they can wreak all kinds of havoc on the body and particularly the reproductive organs, causing things like pelvic inflammatory disease (PID) and secondary infertility.

The best defense against STIs is a good offense, and that means three things: getting tested regularly, practicing safer sex to reduce your risk of infection, and getting vaccinated where possible.

GET TESTED REGULARLY

If you are sexually active, it is a good idea to get a full STI screening once a year. Your doctor can order these tests, or you can go to a clinic like Planned Parenthood that specializes in reproductive health. Sometimes, public health organizations make free testing available, especially for HIV. If you do not have health insurance, or your insurance does not cover STI testing, it may also be possible for you to get inexpensive or free STI testing through your local or regional government's department of health.

Some people may decide to get tested more often than once a year. This can be a good idea if you are sexually active with multiple people, if you engage in sex play with strangers, or if you have a partner who does either of these things. People who are planning a pregnancy (or planning to father a child) should also be tested before they begin trying to conceive.

Other people may decide that based on their relative level of risk, they don't need to get tested every single year. This may be perfectly appropriate. Or it may not: people in supposedly monogamous relationships can and do cheat, and they may lie about cheating. People also lie about STI status. According to Planned Parenthood, about one in three people who have a known STI will lie about their STI status in order to have sex. Adding injury to insult, people don't always know when they are infected. Sometimes people can't inform their partners that there's an infection risk because they have no idea that they are infected with an STI, perhaps because they have had no symptoms.

"I went to the doctor with STD symptoms and he said it was probably just a UTI [urinary tract infection] because 'girls like you' don't get STDs. He gave me antibiotics, and I guess that took care of it, but I still think he should have tested me and told me exactly what was going on. I had had UTIs before and I am pretty sure from the symptoms that I didn't have a UTI."

You can and should get tested as often as you think is right for you. If you should run into a health care provider who dismisses your request for STI testing, remind the provider that STIs are not weight related. If necessary, you can ask for a referral to another doctor, or you can simply go to a reproductive health clinic or specialized STI testing clinic.

PRACTICE SAFER SEX

Most STIs are transmitted through bodily fluids, which include semen, vaginal secretions, and blood. This means that the best way to prevent infection is to prevent contact with those fluids.

The highest risks of STI infection are found in the most common sexual activities: penis-in-vagina intercourse, anal intercourse, and oral sex. Not only do these involve body fluids, but they also involve the tender, fragile mucous membranes that line the vulva, vagina, anus, rectum, mouth, and throat, which means that it is easier to get an infection in these areas.

Fortunately it is very easy to reduce infection risks for these activities. Use a condom for any activity that involves a penis. Use a dental dam—a latex or polyurethane sheet that goes between your mouth and your partner's body—for any activity that involves a mouth in contact with a vulva, vagina, or anus. Put the condom on the penis as soon as it is fully erect to ensure that pre-ejaculate and semen are completely contained. For a quick, easy dental dam, cut the tip off of an unlubricated condom, then cut from end to end along the tube so it can be unrolled into a stretchy sheet. Or try plastic wrap, which is inexpensive and is available in fun colors.

Other sexual activities are generally less risky in terms of STIs. However, there may still be some risk. You can reduce your risks further by using latex or nitrile gloves for penetration using the fingers or hand, avoiding getting anyone else's body fluids on any part of your body where you have cuts or broken skin, and using condoms on dildos, vibrators, or other toys if they have more than one user.

Other STIs, like herpes, are transmitted by contact with a lesion or sore. The best way to prevent these infections is by preventing contact with lesions or sores, which means that taking a minute to turn the lights on and visually check out your partner's genitals before you have sex is a great idea. The same visual check is a good way to make sure you're not exposing yourself to parasites like lice or scabies. You can easily make this part of sex play. It's a good argument for not leaving yourself in the dark.

GET VACCINATED

Vaccinations do not exist for every STI, but the vaccines that we do have provide excellent protection against particular nasty bugs. Hepatitis A and hepatitis B vaccinations can benefit you regardless of your age. HPV (human papilloma virus) vaccination is recommended for women specifically, because of the connection between HPV infections in women and later cervical cancer. HPV vaccination is currently recommended for women under the age of twenty-six.

OW! Preventing Sex Injuries

Love hurts. Sometimes it's the unfortunate collision of someone's knee with your groin, or an elbow with your head. In the heat of the moment, we can inadvertently pinch, whack, shove, and otherwise knock one another around without meaning to. Even kissing can result in unexpected, painful clanking of teeth on teeth or noses on foreheads. Being careful, and trying to pay close attention to what you're doing, helps, but sometimes people move unexpectedly. It happens.

eople also injure themselves during sex in other, more prevent-
ways. Joint and muscle injuries are particularly common and
are particularly relevant when you and/or your partner are fat.

When we get aroused, our ability to feel pain tends to diminish.
The laws of physics, unfortunately, never take a vacation. Heavier
bodies have a lot of momentum and that momentum can be hard to
control. Some of us are not in great physical shape, which makes it
that much more likely for things to get away from us. Even for very
fit people, sometimes, if your alignment is off and/or your muscles,
ligaments, and joints are not strong enough to take the stress, you
can hurt yourself or a partner during sex, quite by accident.

Not only can you hurt yourself, but you may not even notice it
immediately. Some injuries are sharp and unmistakable. But arousal
has a tendency to raise people's thresholds of pain considerably.
Thanks to being aroused, you can sometimes hurt yourself and go
on hurting yourself for as long as the arousal is present, only to come
down and suddenly realize you're in significant pain.

The best way to prevent a sex injury is the same as the best way
to prevent a sports injury: training! Exercise strengthens muscles,
ligaments, and joints throughout your body. You don't have to turn
into a gym rat. Even light exercise can increase your flexibility and
your strength, improve your stamina, and reduce your chances of
getting hurt. This is especially true if you have any known trouble
spots, like bad knees, a bad back, or a repetitive stress injury like
tendonitis. You can do specific exercises that strengthen and help to
stabilize the parts of your body that are weak, possibly with the help
of a physical therapist or personal trainer specializing in injury reha-
bilitation who can teach you techniques to help specific parts of the
body and prevent specific types of damage.

Because sex is a form of exercise, you also want to warm up, if
you can, before you launch into a full-blown "workout." This might
not seem sexy in the abstract, but when you consider that you can put
your arms and legs through a significant range of motion in the pro-

cess of making out, groping, caressing, and helping your partner disrobe, it soon becomes evident that you don't necessarily have to run off for a quick ten minutes of calisthenics in order to warm up your muscles, joints, and connective tissues. Stretching—while bending over to untie your shoes or pull off a stocking—or shimmying out of your clothes also helps. If you feel particularly stiff, though, it's really fine to take a moment to limber up the stiff bits. It sure beats having your sexy encounter interrupted by a yelp of pain.

It can be hard to concentrate on anything other than sensation and pleasure when you're having sex, and in some ways that's as it should be. If you know you are prone to joint or muscle injuries, though, it pays to be attentive to form as well. Try to check in with your body while you are having sex and see whether or not your body is positioned in ways that are well aligned, straight rather than twisted, and not unnecessarily restricted. See whether your knees and hips are moving easily and without a feeling of pain or resistance. Try to make sure, especially if you are thrusting with your hips and/or legs, that your trunk is aligned so that your knees, hips, and shoulders are all facing the same direction. If you are supporting a lot of weight on your hands, you might try putting the weight on your whole forearms rather than just on your hands, to relieve strain on the wrists. Avoid locking your elbows and knees, too, if possible. If something feels out of whack, or like it's taking you a lot more effort to maintain a position or a posture than it should, take the few seconds to reevaluate and to shift position to something that feels better.

If you try to do something strenuous during sex and you hear that little voice in the back of your head protesting, try to pay attention. I know it's not always easy, and things that sound cool and exciting sound even cooler and more exciting when you're all aroused and feeling completely bulletproof. But the sad fact is that if you cannot do a hundred pushups without hurting yourself, having an erection is unlikely to make it possible. If you couldn't do the splits yesterday morning, all that's going to happen if you try it now is that you'll be walking like a cowboy for the next two weeks. Sexual desire is not Magic Badass Juice. Being a little sore the next day is one thing. Ending up in your orthopedist's office clutching a vial of pain pills and scheduling knee surgery is another. Enough said.

Dysfunction Junction

It's all very well to have a book full of advice on how to have a better sex life. But what if the problem isn't a lack of confidence or any problem finding a partner—it's that things just aren't physically working? There are many types of sexual dysfunctions to which the flesh can be heir.

Fat people are not necessarily more likely to suffer from sexual dysfunction than thinner people, but they are definitely more likely to have their sexual dysfunction be blamed on their fatness. This is unfair and unhelpful, and nothing but an easy out for the physician. After all, any idiot can look at you and say, "Ah, you're fat! That must be why!" The visual diagnosis, in this case, is irresponsible: many sexual dysfunctions have distinctive, treatable causes, and they don't generally have anything to do with weight or fatness. Knowing more about these dysfunctions and how they happen can help you troubleshoot, and it can also help you self-advocate for appropriate medical care if you choose to seek it.

There are several broad types of sexual dysfunction, of which the most common are loss of desire, erectile dysfunction, dyspareunia, and vaginismus.

LOSS OF DESIRE

If you used to feel sexual desire on at least a somewhat regular basis, but your sexual desire wanes or suddenly stops, it is called *loss of desire*. (This is distinct from the experience of those whose lack of desire is consistent, which is not necessarily a sign of dysfunction.

People for whom this is true may simply be asexual.) Loss of desire can be psychological: new parents often report losing sexual desire for a while, due to stress, lack of sleep, and new responsibilities. It is a common symptom of depression, sometimes going along with what is called *anhedonia*, the reduced ability to feel pleasure. Traumatic experiences (especially if they are sexual in nature) can cause people to lose desire for significant periods of time. Loss of desire can also be biological—the result of changes in hormone levels or an underlying illness. Endocrine disorders, like thyroid malfunction, can often affect sexual desire. Women may experience loss of desire more frequently than men do, but whether this is due to biological factors or social ones—including the fact that in our society, masculinity is expected to include constant sexual desire—is not clear.

If you believe that your loss of desire is psychological or stress related, just giving yourself some time and space, and not worrying about it overmuch, can help. Talking to a therapist or counselor might also be a good idea. If you suspect that the cause might be biological, or the "relax and wait a while" approach isn't helping, talk to your doctor.

ERECTILE DYSFUNCTION

This is the modern Viagra-ad-friendly euphemism for impotence, the inability for men to get or keep an erection. Impotence happens for many reasons. Sometimes it happens just once or twice and then resolves itself. Other times it is chronic and consistent. Almost all men experience it at one point or another in their lives.

Doctors tend to talk about impotence as being either "organic" (biological), or "psychogenic" (meaning psychological, emotional, or stress related). Some types of biological impotence that have to do with poor blood flow to the penis can be helped with drugs, including Viagra and its relatives. Other types of biological impotence might be caused by smoking (another reason to quit!), neurological problems, or the side effects of drugs, whether prescription or recreational. Alcohol, which is a central nervous system depressant, is notorious for causing impotence.

Psychogenic impotence can come from stress, guilt, fear, worry, or, paradoxically enough, too much excitement. Depression and anxiety disorders often have impotence as a symptom, and traumatic experiences may also include impotence in their fallout.

Psychotherapy or counseling, and possibly working with a sex therapist, can help when being patient and trying to cut yourself some slack doesn't. Viagra and similar drugs will not help psychogenic impotence except via the placebo effect. Save the money you were going to spend on little blue pills and spend it on a therapist who specializes in helping people with sexual dysfunction instead: it's a much more appropriate treatment.

DYSPAREUNIA

Dyspareunia is a catch-all diagnosis that really means "in women, chronically painful penetration." Typically, if a woman has been experiencing painful vaginal penetration (or painful attempted penetration) for six months or more, it is diagnosed as dyspareunia. Dyspareunia, like other sexual dysfunctions, can be psychological or biological in nature, or some combination of the two. There are many biological conditions that can make vaginal penetration painful for women (the Johns Hopkins Dyspareunia and Vulvar Pain Center lists more than forty). Because some of the conditions that can create dyspareunia are quite serious indeed, and also because many dyspareunia-causing conditions can be treated successfully, this is something that should definitely be checked out by a doctor.

If you and a doctor have ruled out a biological origin for dyspareunia, psychotherapy with a sex-positive therapist may help. Some women also have good luck self-educating about sex and arousal by reading, masturbating, and having frank talks with their partner(s) about what works for them and what does not. Since one possible cause of dyspareunia is simple lack of arousal and lubrication, learning more about what arouses you (and paying attention to that when you have sex) and using a good sexual lubricant can help.

VAGINISMUS

Vaginismus means that the muscles surrounding the vagina clamp down whenever one attempts to insert something into the vagina. Women with vaginismus may find it impossible to use tampons or have gynecological exams performed, let alone be penetrated sexually. The causes of vaginismus are often psychological, but not always. Vaginismus could be originally triggered due to some biological problem, illness, or infection that made penetration extremely painful at one time, causing the body to develop the protective reflex to try to close the vagina and prohibit any further penetrations. It may develop due to a traumatic, violent, or abusive sexual history. Many women who experience vaginismus may never actually know why it began or be able to trace it to any particular incident. Fortunately, it is not always necessary for women with psychogenic vaginismus to know why they have it in order to make progress in reducing or curing it.

Some women have success with a DIY treatment for vaginismus that involves a lot of self-education, reading, discussion, and perhaps psychotherapy to find out what helps them feel relaxed and aroused. They follow this up with gentle attempts at inserting something into the vagina—at first something quite small like a pinkie finger, but gradually, with time and patience and lubrication, perhaps something larger like a small dildo. Other women prefer to work with doctors, sex therapists, or psychotherapists in their efforts to overcome vaginismus.

Some women, however, simply decide that they are happier and better off not having to deal with vaginal penetration of any kind and don't worry about it. The only medically relevant argument against doing this is that penetrating the vagina is necessary for standard gynecological health care. If a woman is unable to bear having her vagina penetrated in any way for any reason, pelvic exams will be difficult or impossible, leaving her at risk of being unable to take advantage of early detection methods for cervical and other cancers.

Keeping Your Head When Your Feet Are in the Stirrups

I have yet to meet anyone, regardless of body size or weight, who looks forward to the annual gynecological exam, for the very good reason that there is really nothing about it that is in the slightest bit pleasant. For some of us, the only thing that gets us in the door at all is the knowledge that getting that annual exam might make a huge difference in our health: the earlier cervical and uterine cancers are detected, the better your odds of survival in the long term. So we grit our teeth, perch our naked butts uncomfortably on the end of those narrow exam tables, endure the duck lips of doom, and wait impatiently for the cavity search to be over. All the while, we try our best to retain a mature, even-tempered, reasonable tone of voice while talking with this person who is twiddling a bottle brush in a place where Nature never intended a bottle brush to go.

Being fat can make it even harder to stay calm, cool, and collected at the gyno's, not least because recent research has revealed that doctors' anti-fat prejudice makes them less than likely to be comfortable performing routine gynecological exams on fat women. In an article called "Stigma and Discrimination in Weight Management and Obesity" in the *Permanente Journal,* researchers Kelly Brownell and Rebecca Pugh reported that 17 percent of physicians were reluctance to perform them on fat women, and as many as 83 percent said they were reluctant to perform the exams on women who themselves seemed reluctant about the examination, as many fat women understandably are. In the Big Big Love Survey, although 93 percent of respondents said they had access to adequate routine reproductive and sexual health care, 31 percent of respondents said they had experienced complaints from health care practitioners that it was difficult to examine them properly because of their weight, and 10 percent had been treated disrespectfully or dismissively by medical personnel because of the patients' size.

There's not much to love about the gynecological experience at the best of times, and feeling like your practitioner does not want to deal with a fat patient, or that you are imposing an enormous burden on your practitioner because of your size (you aren't!), makes it all the worse. Here are some tips that will let you help yourself, and help your doctor, be less reluctant, more comfortable, and more likely to accomplish this vital health care screening with the recommended frequency.

INTERVIEW YOUR PRACTITIONER

You can learn a lot—and help them learn, too—by asking your doctor and your doctor's staff whether they are prepared to deal with someone of your size. Ask them if they have dealt with fat patients in the past, and, if you think it is likely to be relevant, whether their chairs, exam tables, and other facilities are large and sturdy enough for someone of your size. You may also want to ask whether there are armless chairs in the waiting area, if armchairs and your hips don't get along very well. Sometimes these things just haven't occurred to them, remarkable as that may seem. Take advantage of the teachable moment.

DECIDE IN ADVANCE WHETHER YOU ARE WILLING TO BE WEIGHED

Being weighed, for some people, is worse by far than any gynecological exam. (I personally experience what I call PTSD—post-traumatic scale disorder—so you're in good company if you say no.) Fortunately, there is no law that says you must submit to being weighed if you don't want to be. It is not a medically necessary part of a gynecological exam.

Besides, your health care practitioner can see that you're fat. She doesn't need a scale to figure it out. Deciding in advance whether you want to be weighed lets you prepare what you want to say about it to your health care practitioners. Usually, a firm, calm "I prefer not to be weighed" is sufficient. If they balk, as they may, you can tell them that if there is a compelling medical reason that they need to know your weight, such as calculating the dosage of a medication, you will be happy to discuss it with them, but otherwise you prefer not to be weighed. Note that if you do choose to be weighed, and you think or know that you weigh more than 300 pounds, you might want to ask in advance to make sure your doctor's office scales will accommodate you. Scales come in a range of weight limits and if you're going to be weighed, it might as well be on a scale that can actually weigh you accurately.

BYOB

That's *bring your own bathrobe* (although I'll be honest—there've been a few gynecological experiences in my life where a healthy snort of bourbon would've been welcome). The paper gowns that are commonly used in many clinics these days are not only flimsy and way too tiny to accommodate many fat women's assets but also fugly as sin, fragile, drafty as only glorified pieces of tissue paper can be, and environmentally wasteful to boot. Do the fashion-forward, eco-friendly thing and bring your own (scrupulously clean, please!) bathrobe with you from home. You'll be much more comfortable and you won't be worrying about how to keep the damn paper gown on when it rips like the Incredible Hulk's T-shirt.

MAKE A LIST

Before you go in to the office, make a list of the things you want to have your practitioner address. If you like, you can make two copies and ask that one of them be placed in your chart. Depending on how long your practitioner is able to spend with you and how many items are on your list, you may require a return visit or visits to address them all, but at least you will have them all written down so you won't forget when you get distracted.

KNOW THE EXAM TRICKS YOUR DOCTOR MAY NOT KNOW

For a variety of reasons, doctors sometimes have difficulty performing pelvic exams on fat women. The exam does not have to be a problem; it's really just a matter of having the right skills and knowing the right tricks.

If you have a prominent mons (the mound of flesh just above your vulva) or carry a lot of fat in your inner thighs, you may need to tell the health practitioner(s) that your flesh can be moved gently to make it easier to see the whole vulva. You can volunteer to be an extra set of hands and do this yourself, if reach is not a problem for you. If this seems a little embarrassing, don't worry: the doctor is likely to be even more embarrassed than you are. You are the one with the insider knowledge here—it's your body, and you know it much better than your doctor does. Your doctor may not realize it's even an option to move fleshy bits around. Being willing and able to help move things around can also help during ultrasounds and other types of examinations.

Practitioners may also be shy about reaching into skin folds. In women with hanging bellies, bimanual exams can be facilitated more easily by having the practitioner simply reach into the under-apron crease with the external hand, in order to put the necessary pressure on the uterus or ovaries so that they can easily be felt and examined by the internal fingers. It may be necessary for you to tell your practitioner that it's okay to do this.

If your doctor is having a hard time seeing your cervix, find out if she is using a metal or a plastic speculum, and what size. Different people's anatomies may work better with specula of different sizes and materials. If you can remember what worked from one exam to the next, it can be useful for you to tell your practitioner and have it added to your chart—the practitioner won't necessarily remember, and it might save you both the trouble of having to go through the whole process of elimination all over again. Also, because fatness does not actually change the size or length of the vagina, there is no truth to the notion that all fat women need to be examined with the largest speculum size.

If your practitioner is using an appropriately sized speculum and is still having trouble seeing things properly, it may be because the walls of your vagina are pressing in between the speculum blades, cutting off the view. Your doctor can take an exam glove, cut off the thumb, cut the tip off the thumb, and place the tube around the speculum blades. Once the practitioner reinserts the speculum, there will be a convenient tube of springy material that will form side walls between the speculum blades, holding the vagina open for better viewing of the cervix. Some practitioners also use a condom with the tip cut off for this, but glove material is somewhat thicker and less stretchy and may provide better results.

In the unlikely but possible event that your doctor claims to be unable to perform a particular exam on you because of your size, ask clearly and directly what the problem is. You know your body better than your doctor does. You may already know exactly what to do to shift position, tilt your pelvis, or what-have-you to make things easier on everyone. If a doctor claims to be unable to perform an exam on a fat person, it may simply be because the doctor lacks the experience and specific technique to negotiate that particular body. The more both you and your doctor can think of an exam as a collaborative event, where you are an active, helping participant, the more likely both of you are to end up with a successful exam.

PCOS

Polycystic ovary syndrome (PCOS) is one of the most common reproductive health disorders in women. It is a complex condition that is not completely understood. It is considered to be primarily an endocrine (gland-related) disorder. One of the chief features of PCOS is that it causes higher than normal levels of androgens (sometimes called "masculine hormones," although all sexes have them) such as testosterone. This in turn causes some of the symptoms, like excess facial and body hair. Other symptoms include not only the ovarian cysts that give the syndrome its name but also other things that are more likely to be noticed by the individual: irregular and/or prolonged menstrual periods, thinning hair on the head, skin discolorations, skin tags, infertility, and acne.

Unlike many other common types of "female trouble," PCOS has a distinctive fat-related component: about 60 to 70 percent of women who have PCOS are fat. Those PCOS sufferers who are fat tend to carry their weight primarily in their bellies and torsos, in the male-typical pattern better known as "apple shape." This appears to be related both to the high androgens associated with PCOS and to the fact that PCOS causes significant metabolic disturbances. Many PCOS sufferers are insulin resistant, which can lead to type 2 diabetes. High blood pressure is another common symptom of PCOS, as are high cholesterol levels and high blood lipids (hyperlipidemia). These things can, if not managed properly, raise the risk of things like heart attack and stroke.

We do not yet know what causes PCOS, but it does have a strong genetic component. If you have a sister or mother with PCOS, chances are good that you may also have it. If you have PCOS and have a daughter, there is a good chance that she may also have it.

Interestingly, PCOS is also one of the most commonly misdiagnosed or undiagnosed reproductive health conditions, despite the fact that as much as 10 percent of the adult female population may have it. This may be partly because so many PCOS sufferers are fat. It is easy, and common, for doctors to blame PCOS symptoms like irregular periods, infertility, excess hair growth, insulin resistance, and high blood pressure on fatness. However, thin women with PCOS have the same symptoms. So do fat women with PCOS who do manage to successfully lose weight, something that is made more difficult than it might otherwise be by the effects of insulin resistance on the metabolism.

Insisting that a patient lose weight is not an appropriate response to a PCOS diagnosis. Fatness does not cause PCOS and weight loss does not cure it. Some women find that weight loss (even small amounts) can help alleviate some PCOS symptoms; others do not experience this at all.

"My PCOS has changed, but it has not actually gotten any better despite medication and losing over one hundred pounds. I still have the full list of classic PCOS symptoms. Some of it is better than it was. My bloodwork looks much better now, but I think that has more to do with the fact that I exercise every day now than anything else. I still have no idea when or whether I will get a period. I'm still insulin resistant. I'm still fat. I'm still hairy. Don't believe it if your doctor tells you that it'll all get better if you just lose weight. It might change things, and some aspects of it could improve, but it won't necessarily go away."

PCOS cannot be cured, but some of the symptoms can be treated. Hormonal birth control pills can regulate menstruation so that periods are more predictable and easier to manage. Insulin-sensitizing drugs like metformin can help to reduce insulin insensitivity. Regular exercise also helps reduce insulin insensitivity and high cholesterol/triglycerides. Some women benefit from androgen blockers like spironalactone, which can help reduce excess facial and body hair as well as some of the other side effects of elevated androgen levels.

Because ovulation is often unpredictable in PCOS women and may not occur at all for some, fertility can present a problem. PCOS women who are trying to get pregnant can often increase their chances of ovulating with drugs like clomiphene (Clomid). Pregnant women with PCOS are more prone to gestational diabetes than women without, and they should talk to their doctors about this so that proper steps can be taken to normalize blood sugar if it gets out of whack during pregnancy. PCOS women who do manage to get pregnant do not necessarily have problematic pregnancies; it is often only conception that presents a problem.

Lipedema and Lymphedema

Lipedema is a medical condition in which fat deposits in a distinctive pattern, from waist to ankles, in the lower half of the body, often creating an exaggerated pear-shaped body. It can be intensely painful and can create major problems for lymphatic drainage (lymphedema), leading to increased potential for infections and other issues. It is found primarily in women and is often misdiagnosed. Doctors, trained to see fat as the enemy, often fail to see lipedema for what it is; they often assume that the woman is merely fat and that if she loses weight, it will all get better.

This attitude can cause active harm to women with lipedema. Perhaps the most distinctive feature of lipedema is that the fat in the lower half of the body behaves differently from other body fat and is virtually impossible to lose. Sufferers who undergo weight loss surgery find that they lose weight from the waist up only; anorexic women can lose virtually all other body fat yet still retain lipedemic fat in the lower body. Attempts to remove this lower-body fat surgically with liposuction have, in general, not helped solve the problem (and in some cases it seems to have created additional ones). "Just lose weight" is therefore not a medically appropriate response to the possibility of lipedema. Weight loss won't make lipedema go away.

Lipedema can be treated, but so far it cannot be cured. Successful treatments include lymphatic drainage massage, the use of elastic bandages and compression garments to help with lymphatic drainage and blood flow, and physical activities like swimming that encourage better circulation. Weight maintenance can help keep lipedema from worsening, in some cases.

Women who have a distinct persistent pattern of fat deposition in the lower half of the body, especially if they tend to lose weight only in the upper half of the body, should discuss lipedema with a doctor.

Lymphedema usually goes along with lipedema, but it can also exist on its own, without lipedema. Unlike lipedema, lymphedema can affect just one limb, or it may affect more than one. Lymphedema is caused by blockages of the lymphatic system and can affect men or women of any size or weight. Lymphedema does not feature fat deposits as part of its normal symptoms in the way lipedema does. However, medical sources agree, although they do not necessarily agree on why this is so or how it happens, that fatness itself can contribute to lymphedema.

Sexually speaking, lipedema and lymphedema can be challenging, to say the least. One of the nicknames of lipedema is "painful fat syndrome." The affected areas can become highly sensitive, and it can be painful to be touched. Given that lipedema affects the body below the waist, this has obvious repercussions for many sex activities.

For both lipedema and lymphedema patients, flexibility and the ability to flex and bend the legs may be compromised by the swelling of the legs and/or hips. This varies from person to person, and some people are naturally more flexible than others. The legs may also feel uncomfortably heavy, and it may be hard for people to hold their legs up in the air for long periods or even at all. Some lymphedema/lipedema patients also experience edema swelling in the abdomen or genitals. How and whether this complicates sex will likely be highly individual and variable.

That being said, there is no reason for lipedema and lymphedema patients to avoid sex. One lipedema patient in her forties, interviewed for this section of the book, said that she thinks sex is good for lymphedema/lipedema in some ways, "because it's exercise for the bottom half, provides some massage that gets lymph moving, and keeps things more supple. It can, depending on position, open up the inguinal lymph nodes a bit." She also spoke in favor of eroticizing the elastic bandages and compression garments that edema patients often wear in order to support lymphatic flow. "I have had sex both while bandaged and wearing compression stockings: bandages make good sex handles!"

Lipedema, specifically, is responsible for a very particular form of the "pear" body shape. The pear shape is often eroticized by fat admirers who like the big butt, hips, and thighs that are its hallmark. People dealing with lipedema may have strong feelings about having others get an erotic charge out of something that is a medical problem and a health concern. On the flip side, some women with lipedema capitalize on its extreme effects on body shape; not a few adult BBW website models clearly show the characteristics of lipedema in the bodies they show off to admiring paying audiences.

Lipedema and lymphedema patients must take special care to avoid injuring swollen tissues, including during sexual activities. Because lymph circulation is poor, the risk of infections and tissue damage is high and recovery from injury or infection takes longer. Pressure, impact, or friction on affected areas can cause damage more easily than it would on a person without edema, so be careful when grabbing, kneading, spanking, slapping, and so on. People who engage in BDSM play need to be especially careful: bondage, flogging, whipping, pinching, restraint positions, and even some types of sensation play involving affected areas may cause significant problems for someone with lipedema or lymphedema.

Gynecomastia

Gynecomastia is enlargement of the breasts in people whose breasts are not supposed to be enlarged—that is, biological males. It has two primary causes: enlargement of the mammary glands, and deposits of fat in the breasts. In some men, both causes can be present simultaneously. Because the breasts are one of the places where bodies deposit fat, fat men in particular often do have noticeable breasts instead of the flat chest that is considered male typical.

Gynecomastia caused by fat is not a disease and does not present health risks. It is really a cosmetic issue. Some men do choose to have their gynecomastia "fixed" with cosmetic surgery, either through the removal of enlarged mammary glands or through liposuction. Like all liposuction, this lasts only as long as the fat stores are not replenished, so it may well end up being a temporary measure.

Gynecomastia does not appear to have any link to the risk of breast cancer. Both biological males and biological females can get breast cancer; the risk is far higher for biological females. Some men who begin to develop gynecomastia, however, are not sure what is going on and worry that they might have cancer. If you experience swelling in your breasts and it worries you, or you aren't sure what's causing it, you should talk to your doctor.

Regardless of whether you ever encounter gynecomastia, lymphedema, lipedema, PCOS, or any of the other health conditions in this chapter, taking care of your body and your health is an important part of your sex life. Few people are capable of feeling sexy and saucy when they feel unwell or are in pain. No body is always healthy—that goes for thin bodies as well as fat bodies. We all get sick sometimes; we all suffer injuries and accidents. But there's no reason to think that because you're fat you have no recourse if you feel unwell. You have every right to do whatever feels appropriate to help yourself have the healthiest body you possibly can, regardless of your size. Looking after yourself with appropriate medical care, good nutrition, pleasurable movement, and restful sleep are all part of taking care of yourself and your health—and, of course, good lovin' never hurt either!

chapter six

Getting Physical

This section is all about making your sex life better, from giving and getting enthusiastic consent to happily getting on top. Whether you have sex only with yourself, with a single significant other, or with a rotating cast of happy playmates, it can be helpful to have some frank and fat-friendly advice, because these logistics do not necessarily come naturally. In this section we get a little graphic and a lot specific, with notes on positions, supports and positioning aids, sex toys, and a wide variety of sexual activities, including a variety of flavors of kink, that can help you find the kinds of adventure you've been wanting—and avoid the kinds you don't. A selection of "Fat Sex Questions Greatest Hits" rounds out this section of practical, hands-on sexy tips.

Yes! Yes! Yes!

In a perfect world, all sexual consent would be fully and completely enthusiastic. Anything less would just not be good enough. Enthusiastic consent is more than just a dull "Oh, okay" or a resigned "I guess I will if you really want to." Enthusiastic consent is exactly what it sounds like: being able to say, as a fully engaged, thoughtful, invested partner, that you know exactly what you're getting yourself into and, yes, indeedy, you really do want to do exactly that!

Enthusiastic consent is an important idea for anyone who is sexually active and, perhaps even more important, for anyone who may be at some sort of social or cultural disadvantage. Because fatness is so vilified, and fat people are so often hated and mistreated, fat people can sometimes end up feeling like they don't actually have much choice when it comes to their sexuality. They may feel as if they don't deserve or aren't good enough to choose to do only the things they really want to do and the people with whom they really want to do them. Other people may try to play on those feelings of worthlessness and of being undeserving to exploit or coerce fat people sexually. When enthusiastic consent is not the baseline for engaging in any sort of sexual activity, it can be easy for people who may not be in a position of power to be mistreated and misused.

How can you make sure that you are giving—and getting—enthusiastic consent? The single most important thing is to have opinions and express them. There is nothing enthusiastic, or even particularly consenting, about a shrug, a grunt, or a sighed "I guess so." If you can't get up any more enthusiasm for sex than you could for, say, going to get your teeth cleaned, why bother? That's not a frame of mind in which you're going to have good sex!

It's okay if you don't want sex right now, or even ever. You don't have to have sex every time the opportunity presents itself. I promise that none of the relevant bits of your anatomy will shrivel up and fall off if you don't have sex. Sometimes you're just not into it. It's totally normal and okay to not always be into it. Other times you might very well be into it, very much so. It's those totally enthusiastic yeses—and the "Oh my god right now!" and "If you don't do me in the next ten seconds I'll probably die" moments—that are what we're looking for here.

The most important thing regarding getting enthusiastic consent is asking for it and listening to the answers. If a partner's reactions are not enthusiastic and engaged, it's okay to stop and ask, "Are you okay? Is what we're doing okay? Is there something else that would be better?" It may be that your partner is tired or stressed out. Or maybe he's been trying to figure out how to tell you that he needs something different from what you've been doing but has been worried about hurting your feelings. Another part of getting enthusiastic consent is paying close attention to what elicits the most heartfelt and genuine positive reactions from your partner. Some people are not very demonstrative during sex, whether by nature or because they have learned to be still and quiet because of a lack of privacy. So it may be that your particular partner is not likely to be the type to shout "Yes! Yes!" when you're doing something he or she likes. But there may be other cues that will provide nonverbal guidance, if you look for them. If you're not sure whether some little noise or movement is the nonverbal equivalent of enthusiastic consent, ask.

Sometimes you will be able to give, and get, enthusiastic consent without a hitch. Other times it will require a little more communication, a little more negotiation, a little more care. This is all as it should be. People are complicated and sexuality is even more so. If you have a little voice in the back of your head saying "But it should all come naturally!" just tell that little voice to go get stuffed. Same thing with any little voices saying "But I should magically know exactly what my partner wants and how to do it or I'm a lousy lover!" or "But I don't want to seem high maintenance because I'm already fat and I can't ask for too much!" None of this is true, and all of it will get you in trouble if you let those beliefs run your sex life. You're much better off concentrating on—and negotiating your way to, when need be—that heartfelt, totally committed "Yes! Yes! Yes!"

Assume the Position

Finding the right position for sex is something that almost everyone struggles with from time to time. People are often needlessly embarrassed by this, thinking that if they were only thinner, fitter, stronger, or whatever, they would never have those awkward sexual moments. It's not true. It doesn't really matter what size you are, how fit you are, or even what kind of sex you have. Differences in heights, body sizes and shapes, degrees of flexibility and mobility, temporary injuries, long-term disabilities, pregnancy, even the types of surfaces you have sex on can all necessitate strategic action. What makes these moments less awkward is remembering your sense of humor and hanging on to the knowledge that it's something that happens to everyone.

There are often numerous possible solutions to any positioning problem. You may need to try quite a few to find the one that works for you. Different types of problems, and different kinds of bodies, will need different tactics. At the same time, there are three general principles that are particularly likely to be of help to fat people and their partners.

BE FIRM

There's more cushion for the pushin' with fat partners, but underneath that cushion (and the pushin') there needs to be a firm foundation. Soft cushions and beds may feel nice, but they are squishy. That means that not only are things more likely to move in an uncontrolled fashion when what's under them compresses, but body parts are also more likely to sink down into the cushion and become harder to get to. Anyone who has ever tried to have sex on a waterbed has found out, probably the hard way, that the genitals are located in the part of the body likely to be farthest below the waterline, which makes them rather tricky to get to. Firm mattresses and cushions, on the other hand, hold you up. They also give you something to push against. So do sturdy sofas, chairs, and other furniture with firmly stuffed, well-constructed cushions. Natural-fiber-filled futons are particularly suited to fat sexy romping, since they are dense and do not compress much.

SEEK SUPPORT

Let's face it: gymnastics are exhausting and, besides, you're having sex—you want to be able to concentrate on sensations and emotions that aren't "if I have to hold this position for one more second my kneecap is going to pop off and fly across the room." Instead of contorting yourself in some uncomfortable and unwieldy way, grab a pillow or cushion and use it to support yourself. Use however many pillows you need, and reconfigure them at will. Firm and dense pillows are better than soft and springy ones for all the reasons outlined above. Many people find that sofa and chair cushions work really well, in part because they are firm and in part because they are large.

A somewhat pricey but extremely functional option is to purchase cushions and supports specifically made for sex. Liberator Bedroom Adventure Gear makes top-rated, high-quality heavy-duty sex supports, pillows, and furniture, including some items specifically sized for "plus size" users (although their regular sizes are fairly generous, and not all fat people would necessarily need to scale up). Many people who use these swear by them. They have been engineered to help people overcome common positioning issues, and so you may find that you require less trial and error to find a workable position for your particular case.

There are also devices available to help hold legs up in the air, with one popular one sold under the brand name Sex Sling. These are basically long strips of wide nylon webbing with a Velcro-fastening cuff at each end. The cuffs go around the ankles, while the middle of the strap (padded, in the deluxe model) can go behind the neck or upper shoulders. You could also DIY your own version of this fairly easily, with a trip to a camping supply store and a little ingenuity.

This would be a good option for very large people who are concerned about having enough webbing for a proper fit, since webbing can be bought in whatever lengths you desire.

MAKE ARRANGEMENTS

Sometimes, body parts have to be arranged just so in order for particular positions to be feasible. For fat people, this can include needing to adjust where and how some of the fat parts of your body lie or hang. Fat rolls and swags cannot always be moved, or moved very far, but sometimes shifting them an inch or two to one side or the other makes a big difference. I like to think of it as fluffing the pillows— it's more comfortable and it gives a little lift to the proceedings. If you have a hanging belly, holding it up, lying on your side so it shifts position, or raising your hips on a cushion so that it falls "back" toward your midsection can give a partner better access to your genitals. This can be particularly useful for face-to-face penis-in-vagina penetration—more so if your partner is also fat. If you have fat inner thighs that are making a particular position trickier than it might be, you or your partner might be able to gently hold the flesh back for the time being. It may seem a little embarrassing, but it's really no different than a woman holding up or moving her breasts around— breasts are made up primarily of fat, after all. (You do know the old joke, right? "How do you make ten pounds of fat sexually irresist- ible?" "Stick a nipple on it.") As any well-endowed woman will be happy to tell you, there's absolutely nothing the matter with adjust- ing your cleavage—wherever it might happen to be on your body.

ROLL YOUR OWN

There is no one true way to have sex. There is no single position that is right. There are no positions that are wrong. You do not get extra points for being able to have an orgasm while simultaneously hang- ing from the chandelier, wearing a gorilla suit, and singing "Bohe- mian Rhapsody." No one except you is going to judge you for using whatever assistive devices, toys, gizmos, gadgets, pillows, props, or whatever else you might decide are useful or desirable. There is not a porn film director poised to yell "Cut!" if you change the script in midstream because you're bored or just changed your mind. And there is no secret Sex Olympics judge waiting to leap out of the bedroom closet to take points off of your overall score because your butt jiggled the wrong way at the wrong time.

If you have in mind some right or ideal way to have sex, get rid of it. What's ideal in your head may not be even remotely close to what would be ideal for your body or for your actual sexual pleasure. Because of this, "ideal" sex turns all too easily into a moving target: when the ideal doesn't actually satisfy, we tend to assume that it must be because we did it wrong, because this or that thing wasn't quite right, and so on. We can invent all kinds of reasons it must be our fault that sex wasn't ideal, and all kinds of things we should've done to do it right. Unfortunately, when we do this, we end up chasing an ideal that changes even as we chase it. When the ideal is something you can never attain but can only chase after, you always feel disappointed and dissatisfied.

The only right way to have sex is the way that works for you and your partner(s). If it makes everyone happy and leaves you all feeling good, you're doing it right. That's the only rule there is.

Masturbation

Masturbation is healthy, educational, natural, and fun. It is a great way to get to know what kinds of sensations you like, and a wonderful way to learn how to have orgasms or have them in different ways. It is guaranteed not to put hair on your palms, give you zits, or make it impossible for you to have an orgasm with a partner. It will, however, help you relieve stress, and it might even improve the quality of your sleep or reduce the severity of menstrual cramps (if you get them). Far from the last resort of the lonely and desperate, masturbation is a normal part of sexuality for people partnered and unpartnered—a reassuring, soothing, and pleasurable thing you can do for yourself to take care of your own needs and wants. It is also a fantastic way to learn more about your own body and responses and what sorts of stimulation work best for you.

Or at least it is when you can do it happily and without difficulty. This sometimes poses problems for fat people. Problems come when either a masturbation method that used to work no longer does, or when issues of mobility and reach make it physically difficult to masturbate.

Sometimes we literally outgrow our masturbation techniques. Women in particular often learn to masturbate while lying on their stomachs, so that their body weight helps create pressure between the vulva and either their hand or a pillow or other object. This is all well and good when you are an adolescent, but it might not work so well when you get older, larger, and heavier—particularly if you get significantly heavier. Putting your arm and hand to sleep because you're lying on them is not helpful. A large belly may mean that you have difficulty pressing your vulva against something underneath you. The simple solution: learn to masturbate in some other position.

I know it seems like a no-brainer, but sometimes people have a really hard time doing this when it comes to masturbation. If you used to masturbate lying on your belly, try it while lying on your back or on your side. It will feel weird at first and you may or may not be able to reach an orgasm in the beginning. Try different things until you find a position that feels reasonably comfortable, and then see if a few weeks' or months' practice doesn't make it feel fully comfortable. Getting to orgasm should be easier as you get more accustomed to the new arrangements.

Masturbating when mobility or reach is at issue is also challenging. Some people do find that when they tinker with positioning, reach or mobility problems can be negotiated. Fat can often move around to some degree. Some people find that if they lie on their side, for instance, they may be able to reach around a large or hanging belly that would create a reach problem if they were flat on their backs or standing upright. Other people find that putting a firm pillow under their butts, raising the pelvis a bit, gives enough of a slope to the abdomen and lower torso to shift fat around and make the genitals easier to reach. But these solutions don't work for everybody. Some fat people may, in fact, find that raising their hips shifts their weight in ways that put too much pressure on their diaphragm and chest, making breathing difficult. You may end up experimenting with several positions that don't work well for you before you find one that does. Or there may simply not be a position in which you are able to masturbate with your hands given your specific reach and/or mobility issues.

Another way to approach reach and mobility problems is by using masturbation toys. Many people who have no reach or mobility problems whatsoever also enjoy these. Options include masturbation sleeves for men, vibrators, and dildos, in addition to a variety of household object "pervertables," like hand-held massage showerheads enjoyed by many women. For men, a masturbation sleeve with a rigid housing, like the high-quality, well-made Fleshlight,

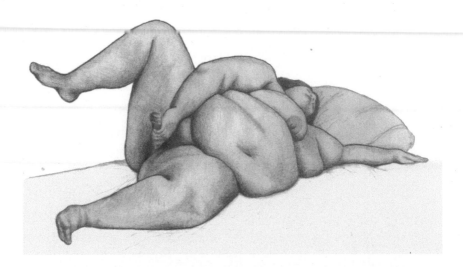

can easily be wedged between pillows or cushions; plus, its long rigid housing gives extra length for holding on to it. Some sex toys, particularly dildos, can also be fastened to smooth hard surfaces with a suction cup device that is sold by many sex toy merchants. These allow you to stick them to a variety of things—think chair seats, bathtub walls, or the top of the washing machine when it's on the spin cycle—rather than having to wedge them between pillows. You can also DIY a more permanent suction cup attachment for the base of many sex toys with a suction cup from the hardware store and some silicone caulk or gasket sealant as adhesive.

For vibrators, the Hitachi Magic Wand, called "the Cadillac of vibrators" by legendary sex toy shop Good Vibrations, has a long handle that makes it useful for many women who have reach issues. It too can easily be wedged between cushions. There are several other longer-handled vibrators available as well, including the Wahl, which is as highly regarded as the Hitachi by many experts. Some long-handled battery-operated vibrators also exist. The Resource Guide has a list of some well-recommended options, and there is further discussion in the "Sex Toys and Accessories" section, page 180.

With regard to dildos, look for length. Don't worry, there's no rule saying you have to insert the whole thing—the additional length is there to give you something to hold on to. Check the Resource Guide for information on reputable sex toy and accessory vendors whose businesses can be counted on to be friendly and accessible for people of size. They can direct you to the long-bodied or long-handled toys they stock.

Penetrative Sex

Penetrative sex is the sexual act most people think of when they hear the words *having sex*. Penis-in-vagina intercourse is traditionally the symbolic central sex act of heterosexuality, and of course it plays a role in procreation if you're interested in getting pregnant the old-fashioned way. However, vaginal and anal penetration really aren't too different from each other in terms of positioning and physics— the two orifices are mere inches from one another in those who have both, after all. For much the same reason, it really doesn't matter whether a penis or a dildo is being used to penetrate. This is why I talk about, and think about, penetration not as a "straight" activity but simply as a human one. It is something that any combination of lovers of any combination of sexes or genders might enjoy, and the positioning advice is just as likely to apply to any two people who engage in it.

As with most other kinds of sexual activity, penetration can sometimes present challenges. Penetration may be difficult or impossible, it may be uncomfortable, it may be hard to achieve in a satisfying way, the penis or dildo may slip out too easily, the demands of topology may make thrusting difficult or uncomfortable once penetration has been achieved, and so forth. These things can happen for a lot of different reasons. Or they may not necessarily happen at all. Every body is different, and every combination of bodies is different, too. It is entirely possible that both partners in a couple can be quite fat indeed and still have no trouble with penetration of any kind. That being said, you may be more likely to find penetrative sex challenging if one or more of the following things are true:

- Both partners are fat.

- One or both partners have a particularly big or hanging belly.

- The partner being penetrated has a particularly big or protruding butt or very thick inner thighs.

- The partner doing the penetrating has a short penis or dildo, or a penis or dildo that is made effectively shorter than it is because of its position relative to a hanging belly.

- One or both partners experience a limited range of leg and/or hip motion.

To find a solution for your particular problem may take some time and experimentation. Refer to the "Assume the Position" section (page 163) for advice on how to approach figuring out worthwhile positions for your needs. Some general ideas follow to help inspire your thinking and play testing.

FACE-TO-FACE PENETRATION

Let's get this out of the way: the classic penetrator-on-top "missionary position" simply does not work well for everybody. And that's okay. This goes for thin couples too, incidentally. The missionary position is vastly overrated. If you find it difficult to let go of the idea that the missionary is the "real" or "ideal" position for penetrative sex, you might find it helpful to know that the historical reason that penetrator-on-top became "the" position for penetration had nothing to do with it being the best or most effective possible sexual position. It was because the Catholic Church deemed that it represented the appropriate relationship between male and female, with the man always above and dominating the woman below him. Still, many people do like the penetrator-on-top position for other reasons, perhaps simply because it's nice to look at each other's faces or because gravity can help make thrusting more intense.

To improve your experience of face-to-face "missionary," try raising the penetratee's rear end on a cushion or other support to help improve the angle of penetration as well as make things more accessible. Another option is for the penetrator to kneel, with the penetratee's legs hooked over the penetrator's shoulders, or to do the same with the penetratee lying on his or her back with their butt at the edge of the bed and the penetrator standing.

Having the penetratee get on top also works well for face-to-face penetration, sometimes better than penetrator-on-top. The penetrator can lie on a bed or the floor

"My favorite position is when my partner reclines on a couch or easy chair and I straddle him on top. It's most comfortable for me and for him, it allows him access to all areas of my body, and me to most of his, and I find it usually works best for me to achieve orgasm."

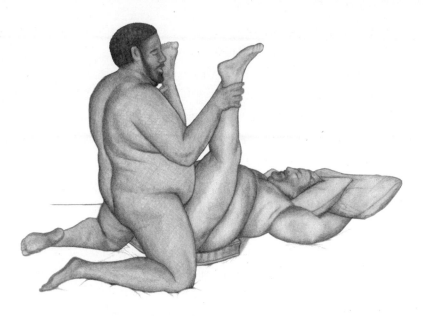

or on some other firm surface, or sit on a chair, sofa, or bench. Picking the right furniture at the right height can help save wear and tear on knees and other joints. Another benefit to trying penetratee-on-top on a chair or sofa is that the person on top can grab hold of the back or arms of the furniture for extra support and leverage.

REAR-ENTRY PENETRATION

Good old doggy style can be hard on the knees, and on the wrists of the penetratee as well, a particular concern in this era of rampant repetitive stress injuries and carpal tunnel syndrome. Bending the penetratee over the edge of a bed or the arm of a sofa sometimes makes a better option. If rear-entry positions are hampered by the penetrator's hanging belly, it may work to lift the belly and rest it on the rear end of the penetratee, a sensation some find erotic in and of itself. The penetrator may also wish to move or shape the penetratee's fleshy rear end or inner thighs to make penetration easier (not too rough, please, and make it sexy!). Rear-entry penetration may work better, in some cases, with the penetrator straddling the penetratee's thighs than it does with the penetrator standing or kneeling between them. Experiment to find out what works best for your particular body, and for the particular combination of bodies you have with any particular partner.

"I sometimes think that if my ass were just a bit smaller, doggy style would be easier. But then, what would my partner grab onto?!"

Spooning-style rear-entry penetration, with both partners on their sides, the penetrator lying behind the penetratee, may or may not be feasible depending on body shapes and sizes. If the penetrator has a big belly or a short penis or dildo, and the penetratee has a very rounded butt, it may simply not be possible to make a connection happen, especially for penis-in-vagina intercourse. Having the penetratee spread her legs, or lift the top leg to allow better access for the penetrator, can make vaginal penetration easier in this position, in some cases. So can changing the angle from which penetration is attempted. Having the penetratee lean forward, pushing the buttocks up and back, sometimes provides a more effective entry.

SIDE-BY-SIDE PENETRATION

There are a number of ways to achieve penetration with both partners lying somewhere between their backs and their sides. People call these positions different things: the *starfish* and the *X* are two names you may come across. The general principle is to let the penetrator and penetratee's bodies intersect at the genitals, arranging everything else so that this can happen most effectively. Try having the penetratee lie on his or her back, and the penetrator lie on his or her side,

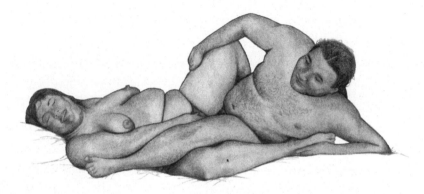

facing the penetrator. The penetratee can put one leg between the penetrator's, and the other leg over the penetrator's hip. This position can be varied to suit your particular comfort and needs. Many people like this position and its variations for penetration because it is fairly low impact and does not put a lot of pressure on joints.

Oral Sex

Oral sex, in general, poses few practical difficulties in terms of positioning. The famed sixty-nine position (mutual simultaneous oral sex) may or may not be possible for any given pair of people, depending on their size, weight, and especially shape. Two big bellies can make it physically impossible to get over the hump, as it were. This may or may not be a drawback. Some people find it extremely difficult to concentrate on giving oral sex when they're being distracted by receiving it. But one-at-a-time oral sex is generally fairly easy to manage, even if one or both partners are very fat.

Occasionally people worry about performing oral sex on fat women. There seems to be a pervasive fear that a fat woman will have an extra-large pussy or labia, and that anyone trying to go down on her will be smothered or suffocated. To me, this has always sounded more like a fantasy masquerading as a fear than it does a realistic worry. In reality, fat women's vulvas are sometimes more fleshy than thinner women's, and sometimes not. Fat women do not have uniformly bigger or thicker labia than thinner women, even though some fat women do have fat deposits in their labia majora and mons. Nor are fat women's vaginas necessarily any larger, longer, or more capacious than thinner women's. There is nothing, in other words, to be worried about. You will not get sucked into the honeypot and be unable to escape.

If you should ever find that getting enough air is a problem when you are performing cunnilingus, just use your hand to gently make some room for better airflow. This works for oral sex with the woman on top just as well as it does when she is lying on her back. If the woman is on top, having a hand in position between your cheek and her vulva is a good precaution anyway, just in case she gets a little carried away and grinds too hard against your face: it is possible to break your nose on someone's pubic bone, but being able to push back can help keep you from harm.

Oral sex on fat men presents few problems, although if the man is on top, straddling the face of the person sucking him, the same hand-by-the-cheek technique can help preserve a clear airway. Alternately, grasping the base of the penis with one hand while sucking also keeps some clear air space, and is something a lot of men enjoy anyway.

Getting on Top

No, you aren't going to crush, smother, suffocate, smash, or other-wise injure anyone you have sex with if you get on top. Cross my heart, hope to die. No, not even if you're honest-to-God super duper fataroonie fatapalooza fat fattity fat. Really. This is the single most common misperception about fat people and sex. It is a question I've been answering for over a decade now, and I have been answering it exactly the same way the whole time. Yes, you can get on top. Yes, I'm serious.

Sure, you could smother, crush, or suffocate someone else with your body: You could take a flying leap onto someone's ribcage and land on them knees first, delivering a punishing two hundred sev-enty four pounds of sternum-cracking fat rage at high speed. You could, presuming you'd somehow made it impossible for them to bite you or fight back, sit on someone's face with a serious vengeance, completely covering their mouth and nose until your implacable *Sitzfleisch* had suffocated the poor bastard to death. Maybe someone should write an action-packed TV show about a fat badass who brings down bad guys doing exactly these sorts of things. (Joss Whedon, I am waiting for your call.)

But these things, I hasten to point out, are not really what most folks would consider sex. Nor are they likely to happen by accident.

Here are the facts: yes, it's possible to injure people during sex. This is just as true for thin people as it is for fat people. But people are pretty robust and resilient, and most folks can take a fair bit of being knocked around without being much worse for wear. Think, for a minute, about the kinds of things that people do for fun—whitewater rafting, riding roller coasters, kickboxing, parachuting, rock climbing, dirt biking, and, for Pete's sake, bungee jumping—and ask yourself whether having a fat person get on top during sex is, even in your fevered imagination, any more likely to be the cause of grievous bodily harm than jumping off a bridge with a rubber band tied around your ankles.

Get on top if you want to, or even if you think you might want to. Do it even if you're a little nervous about it. (You'll be fine.) Do it with care and with pride. Do it slowly; take your time, adjust yourself and your weight so that you are comfortable and your partner is comfortable too. Use a chair back, a headboard, the wall, or what-

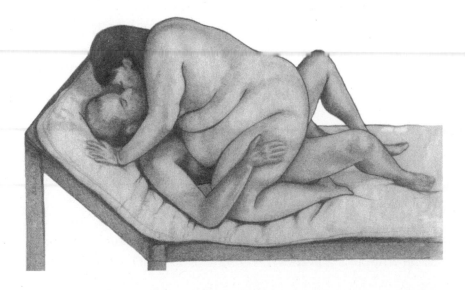

ever is handy to steady yourself and give yourself some extra leverage. Your partner can help with this, too, since she or he has lots of stability from being firmly planted.

Spreading your weight out evenly will be more comfortable for your partner than if your weight is all concentrated in one spot. As with any partner, at any size or weight, watch out for elbows and knees and even for leaning all your weight on one hand when that hand is resting on a soft part of your partner's body or over a joint.

If you need to get off of someone in a hurry, roll off. It's quicker and easier to just roll to one side than it is to figure out how to hoist yourself up off of someone experiencing a muscle cramp or just the normal post-orgasm tiredness.

Don't worry about what you look like. You may be convinced that it's an unflattering angle, but take it from me—the view from below is actually pretty awesome. The important thing is what it feels like. If it doesn't feel good, you can adjust your position, or try something entirely different. But if it does feel good—and it might feel pretty fantastic—you can feel free to rock on with your bad on-top self for as long as you and your partner both like it that way.

Fat Porn and Erotica

In the past, it was often impossible to find any sexually explicit material featuring fat people that wasn't low budget and poorly produced by fly-by-night publishers. A considerable amount of it was overtly shaming or humiliating toward fat women, sometimes in the guise of humor, but sometimes just for the sake of humiliation, a dynamic that spoke volumes about the conflicted emotions the men who made and consumed it must have felt about their attractions to fat women's bodies. Straight fat-admirers who have been in the scene for a while often talk about how as younger men, they had to resort to buying crass, cruel "humor" greeting cards in order to find images of fat women in the nude or wearing lingerie. Sometimes, fat-admiring straight men could find some satisfaction in big-breast genre porn, since large breasts are sometimes accompanied by larger bodies. But in general, fat-related adult material was difficult to find, and, when you could find it, it wasn't very good.

This began to change when *Dimensions* magazine began publishing in 1983. Originally intended to be an adult-oriented fat admiration girlie magazine, it rapidly became a hub for sex-related heterosexual fat community and both sexual and nonsexual connection. *Dimensions* is now exclusively online, and it continues to serve much the same function. Gay male fat-related pornography likewise grew out of its own community. Magazines like *Big Ad*, *Bulk Male*, *Bear Magazine*, and *American Bear*, and a variety of video producers as well, emerged in the 1980s and 1990s to serve gay men who wanted bigger, meatier adult material.

The majority of fat-related adult material, like the majority of all adult material, continues to cater to a male audience (straight and gay). But production values are no longer so low, the business is no longer so uniformly shady, and the furtive and conflicted sensibility that permeated some of the earlier fat pornography is less intense. Part of this is undoubtedly due to the influence of the Internet, which has democratized porn and access to it to a great degree, and part is due to the influence of a new generation of pornographers, many of them women who have dedicated themselves to producing adult material that is size accepting and not quite so relentlessly focused on appealing to the male gaze. This means that, slowly but surely, it is becoming more possible for women (straight and queer), trans people, and men who do not enjoy traditional mainstream porn to find fat-focused adult entertainment they enjoy.

While the mainstream adult film industry continues to crank out dozens upon dozens of boring and more or less exploitative "plumper" and BBW films, there is more interesting and rewarding fare available too. Porn actor and pornographer C. J. Wright, for example, is a genuinely enthusiastic fat admirer whose career seems to combine work and play. BBW model and porn star April Flores, who delightfully describes her dress size as an "extra-medium," works both with her husband, the celebrated photographer Carlos Batts, and with other producers, photographers, videographers, and artists in a variety of media. The creator of the popular pansexual, body-diverse porn site Nofauxxx.com, Courtney Trouble, is likewise an unashamedly fat, sexy entrepreneur who has devoted a career to making more diverse, more interesting, more body-affirming adult entertainment. Numerous BBW, bear, and chub cam-girls and cam-boys and models run their own businesses in which they are the owners, the operators, and also the models. Feminist, lesbian, and queer pornographers like Fatale Media and S.I.R. Video, have also explored a more diverse palette of bodies in their films.

For those who prefer their adult entertainment a bit less explicit, there are other options. Photographer Substantia Jones, who produces the renowned size-positive photoblog Adipositivity, and Molly Bennett, proprietor of Fat Bottom Boudoir photography (and the cover photographer for this book!), are among many exploring a more artistic, but still very sexy and sensual, approach to depicting fat bodies. Some pinup artists, like Les Toil, known for his BBW "Toil girl" renditions of women from the size positive community, focus exclusively on big women. Prose erotica featuring larger bodies can be found in a variety of the contemporary women-oriented erotica anthologies put out by publishers like Seal Press and Cleis Press, which brought out the anthology of fat-positive erotic fiction I edited in 2001, entitled *Zaftig: Well Rounded Erotica*. In addition, at various times, sexy fat 'zines from the queer women's community (like the late, lamented *Size Queen* and *FaT GiRL)* have emerged and then faded out again. Who knows what will emerge next? Only one thing is for sure: fat-positive adult entertainment is very much a DIY field. The next big thing in size-accepting porn or erotica—pun very much intended—could even be you.

Sex Toys and Accessories

Sex toys are a bit like dessert. You don't need sex toys to have a full, satisfying, delicious sex life, but they can be a fun addition. Sex toys can be used solo (see "Masturbation," page 166) or with a partner, and at any time during a session of sex. They can be used simultaneously with other types of stimulation, for instance using a dildo to penetrate someone while you perform oral sex on them or using a vibrator on the clitoris to enhance penis-in-vagina intercourse. Or sex toys can be used all by themselves.

Sometimes people get intimidated or put off by sex toys. Men, especially, are sometimes afraid that if their female partners get used to vibrators, or to dildos that are bigger than the men's own penises, their own flesh and blood bodies won't be good enough anymore. This is unlikely to happen. The fact that you like brownies doesn't mean you don't also like strawberries; your love for a big juicy steak doesn't mean you don't go just as completely gaga over big juicy tomatoes. They're different things, and you can like them all.

It helps reduce the freak-out factor if you think of sex toys as being exactly what they are: tools. These just happen to be tools that let you sexually stimulate yourself or another person in ways that you might not be able to do without them. They simply provide options beyond what you can do all by yourself. The human body, after all, has some built-in limitations to how it can bend and stretch, how many organs it has of any given type, and where body parts are located relative to one another. Sex toys can help you bypass some of these limitations and expand your options.

If you use sex toys with a partner, there are no real barriers to using whatever sex toys turn you and your partner on. If you are using them for masturbation, certain sex toys might be more useful than others, depending on individual mobility and reach (see "Masturbation," page 166). But generally speaking, sex toys are universal and your body size won't have much bearing on your options.

Two arenas where this may not be true are wearable vibrators and dildo harnesses. Wearable vibrators are small, usually "bullet" style vibrators that are designed to be worn by women, with a harness of some sort that holds the vibrator over the labia near the clitoris. The idea is that you can wear them under your clothes and enjoy secretly getting your buzz on with no one the wiser (although, given the fact that most people's crotches don't normally buzz, you might want to try this somewhere fairly noisy). Reviews on these items are mixed: some women love them; for others they really don't get the job done. They can present an additional issue for fat women: these harnesses are produced in the infamous "one size fits all," which, as we all know, usually doesn't. If the harness doesn't fit you, you can seek out fabric webbing at a fabric store or camping goods shop and cut your own straps to whatever length you need. Depending on your shape and how you carry your weight, you may have to adjust the straps significantly in order to bring the vibrator to bear on the right part of your vulva. If this seems like too much of a pain, and it well might, you can also consider sewing a little pouch into the crotch of a tight-fitting pair of underpants to achieve the same goal. Or, if you are blessed with juicy fat labia, you may be able to just tuck the bullet vibe in between and have your own body hold it in place for you.

Dildo harnesses can be had in a range of larger sizes. Several manufacturers, including, notably, some of the most mainstream mass-market brands, make dildo harnesses in "plus size" versions. How big "plus size" is varies considerably. Stormy Leather's "Crown" harness fits up to a 40-inch waist and 60-inch hips; Sport Sheets "Divine Diva" model will go up to 82 inches in the waist. (See Resource Guide for more details.) If you can find a dildo harness that does not force you to wear the dildo directly over your pubic bone, so much the better. Wearing the dildo higher

"I've noticed that as my labia and mons pubis and all that stuff has gotten fatter, I can stick my bullet vibrator on my clit and even if I get up and walk around, it will stay there without me having to hold it. I know that sounds silly, but I LOVE that. Yay for fat pussies!"

up can make thrusting a little less taxing. This is even true if you have a hanging belly. Wearing a dildo on the leading curve of a hanging belly instead of directly over the pubic bone may feel silly at first, but it stops seeming silly the instant you realize how much thrust and control it provides and how it eliminates the problem of a hanging belly getting in the way of easy penetration.

An alternative to conventional dildo harnesses is the thigh harness. Strapping a dildo to your thigh provides new options in terms of positioning and can be much easier on the lower back and other joints and muscles that may be weak or injury-prone. Thigh harnesses also let you put a lot of power behind your thrusts—legs are

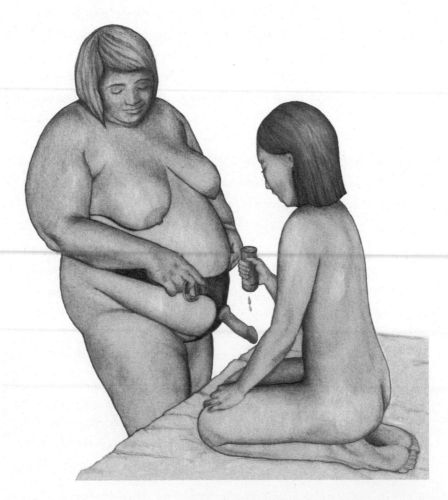

often stronger than lower backs. Frequently thigh harnesses are made of neoprene, the same material as wetsuits, which is stretchy but not wildly so. They usually have a hook and loop fastener. To make them larger, you can make an extender out of a piece of neoprene or sturdy non-stretchy fabric (such as heavy denim or canvas) the same width as the thigh harness band, and use fabric glue to attach more of the hook and loop fastener in appropriate places. Depending on your measurements, and those of the thigh harness you choose, you might also just buy two and connect them.

Double-ended dildos are a little trickier. While there are some fat folks who swear by them, they do not always work out well. One of the chief problems of double-ended dildoes for users fat or thin is that the vagina does not open toward the front of the body. The free end of any straight-bodied double dildo inserted into the vagina is, therefore, going to be pointing roughly toward the knees of the person into whose vagina it is inserted. (Double-ended dildos are typically not recommended for anal use, since they often lack the flared base that would make them safe anal toys.) Although many double-ended dildoes are bendy, it's not necessarily enough to make using them any less awkward or unsatisfying. Some double-ended dildoes, such as the popular Nexus dildo, are shaped with a bend in the middle to prevent this problem. These are less unwieldy, but they come with the same problems as any dildo worn over the pubic bone: a hanging belly may still get in the way. Additionally, for people with reach issues, a double-ended dildo may be impractical as a couple's toy, but the additional length may make them useful for masturbation.

Beyond Vanilla

The saying goes that there are only two kinds of people: people who believe that there are only two kinds of people, and people who know better. The same is true of sex. Many people talk about sex as if there were only two kinds, "normal" and "kinky." This is not a particularly useful distinction, since what an awful lot of folks really mean when they say "normal sex" is "the kind of sex I like" and what they mean when they say "kinky" is merely "the kind of sex I find undesirable."

Human beings enjoy a big spectrum of sexual activities, and each has its fans and detractors. Some activities have a very wide appeal; others are only of interest to a small number of folks with specialized tastes. Beyond the usual range of activities that constitute "sex" for most people most of the time—oral sex, penetrative vaginal and anal sex, masturbation—there are some sexual activities that are sometimes called "kinky" that are relevant specifically to fat people and those who have sex with fat partners.

FAT FROTTAGE

Frottage is rubbing, usually rubbing of the genitals against some non-genital part of the body. Dry humping is one form of frottage that many people know well. Some people also get great pleasure out of rubbing their genitals against, or between, the fat swells and rolls of a partner's body. Mechanically, this is not so different from breast frottage, or tit fucking. However, breasts and fat rolls have different connotations and different emotional resonance, so people may react to it very differently indeed. Tip: If you engage in fat frottage, use a good lubricant to avoid abrasion.

FACE SITTING OR QUEENING

Some people find it enormously satisfying to have a partner "sit" (usually more like squatting) on their face, engulfing their entire face in the vulva or buttocks. Fat partners may be especially sought out for this because of their size, weight, and fleshiness. Face sitting does not necessarily mean oral sex, although it may. Some face-sitting fans like to feel as if they are being suffocated, which may be worrisome for the person doing the face sitting. This sensation can, however, be safely enjoyed for very brief periods (not more than twenty or thirty seconds is a good general rule). Tip: If you engage in face sitting, make sure you have a sturdy support to help the sitter stand back up (or otherwise get off) easily and quickly. A brief flirtation with feeling suffocated might be sexy; the real thing, not so much.

BDSM

BDSM is a portmanteau acronym that stands for *Bondage and Discipline, Dominance and Submission, and Sadism and Masochism*. In practice, it includes all these things and many other variations on the general theme. What they all have in common is either a focus on explicit power dynamics or roles or a focus on sensations that are not necessarily part of more mainstream sexual activity.

Some BDSM practices are the classic whips-and-chains sorts of scenarios most people associate with the term. For instance, a top (dominant) might tie up his bottom (submissive) in bondage, and then spank or flog the bottom. But other BDSM practices look very different. For instance, a dominant might instruct her submissive to do the dishes and polish her boots, something that does not seem sexy to many people but which for some dominants and submissives would definitely be part of their erotic dance together.

Some people include genital sex as part of BDSM. Other people don't. The cliché of BDSM is that it involves pain, but not all BDSM activity does. There is no one way to practice BDSM, and there is no one kind of sexual or erotic activity that "is" BDSM.

Because BDSM sexual practices are so varied, and the ways people enact their BDSM play run such a wide gamut, this book cannot really hope to provide even an overview. If you are looking for good basic information about BDSM, including how-to and other practical information, please see the "Special Issues Sex Information and Education" section of the Resource Guide.

There are some particular places where BDSM and fatness intersect. These may or may not be covered—or even mentioned—in the BDSM literature.

THE SUBMISSION QUESTION

A question that may come up for some fat people interested in BDSM is whether an urge to be sexually submissive is coming from a healthy place. In our fat-hating culture, many fat people grow up and come into their adult sexuality in a psychological environment that treats them as second-class citizens. They may learn that if they are fat, their own sexual wishes don't matter and they should be grateful for whatever they can get. Or they may be conditioned to believe that no one will really want to give them pleasure because of their fatness, and that their sexual role should be limited to giving pleasure to others. Sometimes fat people are taught to think that fat bodies only deserve punishment. And unfortunately people, regardless of size, sometimes learn to link sexuality with bad or abusive treatment because this was what their formative experiences taught them was normal.

Because fat people are at particular risk for these kinds of experiences and for internalizing these kinds of messages, they should also be thoughtful and careful about their urges to be sexually submissive in a BDSM context. No one deserves to be treated badly or abused because they are fat. No one should be limited to only providing pleasure to others because they are fat. No one should have to accept being treated or touched in any undesired ways in order to get attention, love, or sex.

There are lots of psychologically and physically healthy reasons that someone might want to be submissive. Many people like it simply because it means they don't have to call the shots for a while! Making sure that you are submitting for healthy, positive, pleasure-filled reasons is good for your body, your mind, your relationships, and for your dominants, who, if they are ethical and sensible, are also caring people who want you to be as happy as you possibly can.

It's wise to be wary of dominant and sadistic urges, too, since we're on the subject. Any time you might be in a position to harm someone who is vulnerable, it's a good idea to make sure you're in control of your emotions and actions and that you are acting responsibly in an overall context of respect, informed and enthusiastic consent, and care.

EXPLICITLY NEGOTIATE THE FAT ISSUE

Some fat kinksters actively enjoy making fat and fatness an explicit part of their BDSM play. Others do not. Fatness, like race, class, gender, ethnicity, and other issues of personal identity, can be emotionally complicated and volatile. Not everyone is comfortable with playing with these issues and concepts, and even those who are comfortable often have serious limits regarding what kinds of play are okay and what are not. It is not okay to simply presume that a fat person is going to be comfortable with references to fat, fatness, weight, or weight loss. It is also not okay to use these issues as tools for humiliation or "discipline" unless you have specifically and explicitly negotiated this with the person in question. This includes the use of words like *fatty*, *cow*, and other derogatory terms. Whether you are a top or a bottom, you do not have to accept any of this in the context of BDSM play unless it turns you on. If you have not explicitly negotiated the use of such words, or the use of fatness or fat talk in your BDSM play, err on the safe side and don't use them.

YOUR SIZE IS YOUR BUSINESS

It is never okay for a person to demand or insist that a partner or playmate change his or her body—either gaining weight or losing it—for a partner's sake. This includes demands that a partner change body size to "prove their love" or as a condition of continuing a relationship. Your body is your business, and what happens to your body, including any attempt to change your body size, is a decision that you should only make yourself for your own reasons.

WEIGHT AND BONDAGE

Fat people can be a lot of fun to put into bondage for the same reason that fat women look sensational in corsets—there's plenty of plush flesh to squish around, mold, and shape. It produces exaggerated effects you just can't replicate with bodies that don't have as much material to work with. For the most part, fat tissues are pretty robust, assuming there are no issues with edema, so bondage by itself is unlikely to cause any special problems for a fat person.

However, some forms of bondage put a lot of stress and strain on particular joints, and doing them on a fat person may put substantially more stress and strain on those joints, causing damage in the process. Any bondage that hyperextends joints or pulls limbs tightly should be done carefully and checked frequently. Suspension bondage may be inadvisable in any form, depending on the weight and the physical condition of the bottom. Pay attention not only to whether joints are under too much strain, but also whether or not the bottom can breathe easily. Some positions will compress the torso or shift a lot of body weight onto the diaphragm and chest, which can make breathing difficult. Stress positions, too, have to be considered very carefully and chosen wisely. Kneeling can be problematic, particularly if it is prolonged, as can being on all fours.

If you are the bottom in a bondage or stress-position situation, be sure you have negotiated a safe word (or other signal) and don't be shy about using it. Remember that arousal can push your threshold of pain a lot higher than it normally would be and that you can end up getting hurt even though you didn't think it was anything serious at the time. If something twinges or feels funny or weird, consider stopping anyway: it's better to check in, adjust, and resume than it is to have to nurse an injury later on.

TAKE CARE WITH SKIN FOLDS

Skin folds and creases can be particularly tender, sensitive, and delicate. Any play that involves this skin should take the potential fragility of the tissue into account. If the skin does become traumatized, abraded, bruised, or broken, keep an eye on it in case of infection. Skin folds can also collect and trap liquids. Be extremely aware of this if you play with hot wax or engage in fire play, because severe burns can result if molten wax or burning alcohol collects in the enclosed space of a skin fold.

Fat as Fetish

Some people who are attracted to fatness are attracted in a very specific way to fat itself. People who fetishize fat are sexually attracted to fat, and the fat parts of fat bodies, in the same way that foot fetishists are attracted to feet. A *fetish*—technically a *paraphilia* in psychiatric terms, since *fetish* is reserved for inanimate objects—means that the foot, or the fat, is an erotic object all by itself. Although people with paraphilias vary on this score, this may mean that the fetishist is less interested in the person whose fat (or foot) it is than in the fat itself.

Being a fat admirer—someone who is attracted to fat people—is not the same thing as being a fat fetishist. Some fat admirers are also fat fetishists, but certainly not all, and the majority of fat admirers do not fetishize fat. One indicator of this is that, of the respondents to the Big Big Love Survey who reported being attracted to fat partners, only 16 percent said they were specifically attracted by fatness itself, and only a small subset of those people would qualify their attraction to fatness as being an actual fetish.

> "I love my partner using my creases and folds to fuck. I love him holding onto my fat thighs and rubbing himself against my leg. I love him wanting to feel my weight on him. I enjoy squashing him, trampling him, sitting on his face and restricting his breathing. There's so many things I can do that a slim woman cannot do. There's so many bits of my body that a slim woman doesn't have. I feel empowered and sexy because of this."

Fetishizing body parts and traits is fairly common in human sexuality. Fat is only one of a large number of bodily features that people can and do fetishize. Other common ones, in addition to feet, include hands, skin color, hair, and noses (interestingly, a fixation on particular types or shapes of genitals is not considered out of the ordinary). No one knows, scientifically speaking, why or how these kinds of highly focused erotic interests form, and people's own explanations of how they perceive their fetishes to have originated vary widely.

Because our culture's party line is that fat is unerotic, ugly, unhealthy, and bad, the fetishization of fat is often seen as particularly outrageous or perhaps as a sign of some sort of mental illness. This is not actually the case. Certainly a fetishist may also have a mental illness—clinical depression, for instance, is awfully common in the general population—but there is no real substance to the idea that having a fetish constitutes a mental illness in and of itself.

The big concern with any fetishistic interest in other people's bodies is with the interactions between the people who have the fetish and the people whose bodies are fetishized. Sometimes people with paraphilic interests can seem creepy or strange because of their focus on a body part rather than a person. If their social skills are not top notch, they are likely to be perceived as obsessive and selfish and as caring not about the person they fetishize but only whether they'll get to satisfy their fetish interests. Fetishists who do not communicate the nature of their fetishes well, and who do not take the time to explain what they want and make sure their partners are okay with that, are likely to offend or at the very least confuse their partners.

"When I was a little girl my mother sent me to a diet doctor and one of the things the doctor did was to measure my fat all over my body with a pair of calipers. They were cold and pinched, and it was very humiliating. I was on a date with a man once who asked how I would feel about letting him touch my fat and all I could think about was that doctor and the calipers. Brr."

Sometimes, a fetishist will encounter someone who is as erotically interested in having part of their body fetishized as the fetishist is interested in fetishizing it. This is rare, but it's also more or less the ultimate fetishist dream.

Much more likely and common is that a fetishist's interest in the fetishized body part is something that doesn't do anything at all for the other person, aside from whatever pleasure they get from their partner's enjoyment. Fetishists who are caring and ethical will do what is necessary to make sure that their partners do not feel neglected. This caretaking can take many forms. It is not necessary for every fetishistic relationship to be a mutually erotic one—sometimes they aren't, by mutual agreement.

From the perspective of the person whose body is being fetishized, fat fetishism can be exhilarating or terrifying or repulsive or bizarre or many other things. Emotions tend to run high where fat is concerned. Some fat people adore being objectified and fetishized. But other fat people have had strongly charged experiences involving other people's objectifying treatment of their fat bodies.

This is not improved by the fact that many fat people, even those who have good body image and are not at war with their fat, simply do not find fat erotic and may be hard pressed to understand why someone else would. Other people simply aren't interested in the idea of having an erotic interaction that is so one sided. It can feel weird for some people to have a partner getting off on something when they're not, and all the more so when what a partner is getting off on is part of one's actual body.

The intimacy issue, with regard to fat, can also be considerable. Because fat and fatness are so emotionally charged, allowing

"Oh man. The first time someone approached me with a fetishy attitude about my fat I freaked out, but later I thought, 'You know, it might be interesting to find out what that's about.' So the next time it happened I decided to make myself available and open to it, and I had a great time! Partly it was fun because the guy had a great sense of humor. He realized how absurdly one-sided the interaction was, and he did his best to make sure I had a good time anyway, which I did. I saw him a half-dozen times and grew to love the totally focused adoration of my body. He was just so into it! Totally kid-in-a-candy-store. I didn't get off on it. But I really enjoyed it. It was kind of adorable in a weird way."

someone even to look at, let alone touch or handle or otherwise interact sexually with, the fat parts of one's body can represent a deep level of intimacy and trust. Creating that kind of trust and intimacy takes time and investment in personal connection. Responsible fetishism takes this into account with a willing and gracious attitude, and it does not merely frame other people as an unavoidable inconvenience that you have to put up with in order to get to the body part(s) that you fetishize.

Feederism

Feederism, also known as the feeder/feedee fetish or encourager/gainer fetish, is an extreme fringe sexual fetish practiced by a very small portion of the population of fat people and fat admirers, themselves already a minority. A nutshell description of feederism is this: feeders or encouragers are people who find the idea or the reality of someone eating excessively and/or gaining weight to be erotic. Feedees/gainers are people who find it erotic to be fed or eat excessively and/or to gain weight. Feeders and feedees may enjoy these things solo—eating or gaining weight on their own—they may enjoy them only with a partner, or they may enjoy them either way.

It is difficult to say for sure how many people have an erotic interest in feederism (or, as it's sometimes called, *feedism*). It's even more difficult to say how many people actually practice it in some form. It's not, by a long shot, a mainstream sexual practice. Nor is it a practice that shelters under the typical BDSM or "kink" umbrella, despite the fact that the power dynamics in feederism often have strong dominant/submissive overtones. The vast majority of fat people, to say nothing of the mainstream population, find it—at best—difficult to imagine or understand. More often, people consider it to be offensive, even horrifying.

It's easy to understand why. Of all the things fat people and their partners could possibly do sexually, feederism is the one that flies hardest and most violently in the face of everything that our culture believes about what is sexy, what is sexual, and especially what constitutes health and personal responsibility. To our fat-phobic culture, the idea that someone would desire and eroticize excessive eating or weight gain is heretical.

For precisely these reasons, as well as the accompanying difficulty of finding partners who share the interest, many people who participate in the feederism fetish do so solely within the realms of fantasy and fiction. Many other types of fetishists who eroticize things that in real life would be ethically or physically problematic do the same thing.

Other people who fetishize feederism develop responsible ways to playact the fetish that are erotically satisfying but are also safe, sane, and fully consensual. Feeder/feedee or encourager/gainer relationships that work on this model allow the person who is eating and/or gaining weight to call all the shots, and to eat exactly as she or he wishes and maintain whatever weight he or she desires. In some cases these relationships do not include truly excessive eating or any weight gain at all: half a dozen doughnuts, a bit of playful sexy patter ("Oh, this doughnut is so fattening but I just can't help myself!"), and a pair of too-tight blue jeans can provide all the erotic eating/gaining stimulation that is desired. There are many ways that people who participate in feeder fetish play can do so ethically and responsibly.

"My boyfriend is into erotic weight gain, and sometimes we talk about it while we are having sex. For instance, if we were having sex and I was on top, I might say something like 'Imagine what it would feel like if my boobs just started growing against you right now, and got so big that they touched the pillow,' and he loves it. I like it too, I like the aspect of growing, but I find a lot of erotic weight gain stuff really creepy, especially when it comes to feeding tubes or immobilization. I like it as a light fantasy, and nothing else."

There is also the potential for abuse with feeder fetish activity, just as there is the potential for abuse with any other form of sexual activity and any other form of relationship. It is never okay for a partner or playmate to demand or insist that another person change his or her body—either gaining weight or losing it—for the partner's sake. This includes demands that a partner change body size in a "prove your love" scenario or as a condition of continuing a relationship. Your body is your business. Anyone who attempts to compel another person to alter his or her body or body habits in any manner that person does not personally wish, is committing abuse. This is true regardless of whether the change is compelled through emotional blackmail, physical violence, threats of abandonment, or any other means.

This very much includes emotional coercion that employs fat acceptance rhetoric. Attempts to convince a person that true fat acceptance or size acceptance means that someone should desire to become bigger and bigger, or that if a person truly loved him- or herself as a fat person, becoming fatter would be no problem, are abusive and wrong. Such statements are a reprehensible and exploitive twisting of the size-acceptance message.

"My first husband got into feederism and wanted to turn me into his first 'project.' Divorce followed shortly."

What genuine size acceptance teaches is that all people and all bodies are valuable and precious regardless of their size or weight. Bigger is not necessarily better—or worse—it is only bigger. Genuine size acceptance means not only making sure that all people have complete autonomy over their own body decisions, no matter what their size or weight, but making sure that predators and unethical people don't use size acceptance as a way to exploit and harm people who may be emotionally, socially, and perhaps physically vulnerable.

Because it is extreme by our cultural standards, because of the potential for abuse, and because it pushes so many buttons regarding sexuality, excess, control and the lack of it, health, disability, and personal responsibility, feederism is the single fat sexuality topic most likely to completely derail all other discussions of fat people and sex. The mainstream press periodically rediscovers it, and, each time it does, it lapses into a frenzy of sensationalist pearl-clutching. In a way that would please the most extreme feeder, media hysteria magnifies the feederism issue into something far, far bigger than it is.

In this way, feederism and public discussions of feederism are a red herring. They create alarm and controversy that derail the ability to have more meaningful and substantive discourse about fat people and sex. All fat people's sexuality, and all fat admirers' sexuality, gets lost in the shadow of the mainstream media's voyeuristic fixation on the feederism freak show. This is a loss and a shame. Hysteria over feederism means that all of us fat people and fat admirers have to fight that much harder to be seen and acknowledged as happy, healthy, functional, normal sexual beings by a society that is already suspicious of fat in all its forms.

> "My current partner is a feeder/ encourager. I've gained over one hundred pounds in this relationship. I miss what I used to look like. At first 'fat and happy' felt like an excellent antidote to my previous partner's controlling behavior; now it just feels fat, and I miss how my body used to move and feel."

Fat Sex Questions Greatest Hits

Since the first version of *Big Big Love* was published in 2000, I have fielded many questions from readers and others about their various problems and concerns with regard to sex and fatness. The following are the six questions asked most often, presented in the hope that they might help answer some questions for this generation of *Big Big Love* fans too.

Q: *I don't have orgasms and I think it's because I'm fat.*

A: If you're having difficulty having orgasms, or have never had one, it could be due to a lot of different factors, but fat is not likely to be one of them—at least not directly. There is simply no real way that fatness, all by itself, can impede the physiological ability to experience an orgasm.

It may be that fatness is indirectly contributing to your orgasm trouble, though. If you are preoccupied by your weight or your appearance, it can be difficult to let yourself feel physical pleasure or concentrate on it enough to reach orgasm. If you are unable to stop focusing on feelings of disgust or hatred of your body, or on what you fear a partner might think of it, then you are unlikely to be able to focus on what you are feeling physically and whether or not it is turning you on and getting you off.

If this is the case, your best path toward learning how to have orgasms lies not in losing weight—because believe you me, some thin women have the exact same obsessions and fixations as you do, and they get in the way of orgasm just as badly for them as they do for you. Instead, the cure is in a combination of learning to accept your own body as it is in the moment and learning how to focus on what turns you on, what feels good physically, and what kinds of stimulation seem to give you the most bang for your buck.

Q: *My partner and I are both fat, and it seems like our bodies are just incompatible for penis-in-vagina intercourse. We've tried everything we can think of and we haven't been able to make it happen. What to do?*

A: I'm sorry you've been dealing with so much frustration. That's no fun. But kudos to you for keeping at it! In many cases, persistence ends up being the critical ingredient. Sometimes a given pair of bodies really are not shaped in ways that make penis-in-vagina intercourse easy, but, if you experiment enough, you can find a way to make it work. Don't overlook the options of holding some of your fat rolls or folds up, or moving them to the side. Sex in water—a hot tub or pool—can also help, between the buoyancy that helps lift fat up and the weightlessness that allows freer and easier movement.

It may help to consider the problem not from the standpoint of working within standard sexual positions, but from the standpoint of achieving only the most critical bit of the union first. If you focus solely on the goal of getting penetration to happen without regard for how it happens, it may free up your imagination in terms of how your bodies might be positioned in order for that to take place. Unfortunately, without seeing the two of you, I can't suggest specifics—I just can't know what factors are causing the trouble. It might help to review the "Assume the Position" section (page 163) to see if there's anything there you haven't already experimented with.

It may be that you two are not able to make penis-in-vagina intercourse happen right now. I understand that this might be a big blow for a lot of reasons, and I'm sorry. As you've probably already discovered, it doesn't have to be the end of your sex life together. There are lots of other ways that people share sex and pleasure and you should absolutely take advantage of all the ones that appeal to you. At the same time, I want to encourage you to keep trying penis-in-vagina sex so long as you are both still interested. You don't have to drive yourself crazy with it, just revisit the territory now and then to see if there is any change. Bodies change, and sometimes what was impossible before can become possible later on.

Q: *I don't want to sound racist, but it seems like the only men who are interested in big women are black or Latino or Middle Eastern or something. What gives?*

A: This is a complicated question to answer. Part of why it's so complicated is that it's a complicated conclusion you are drawing. What you're really saying is not that "only nonwhite men are interested in big women" but "the only men who I notice being overt about their interest in big women are nonwhite men." That's a big difference.

In truth, men of all skin colors and ethnicities like fat women. That much I can say with absolute certainty.

Beyond that, I can only talk about generalities and likelihoods. What I am about to say will not apply to every man, regardless of his skin color or ethnicity. Individual cases will always vary. But there are some general dynamics in Western culture that are probably relevant to the patterns you have noticed about which men are likely to openly express an interest in fat partners and which men are not.

First, there are subcultures where it is more socially acceptable for men to express an interest in a woman who is not slim and cultures where it is less so. Mainstream Western culture (which is to say middle-class, white culture in North America) in the present day does not embrace the idea that plump or fat women might be considered sexually appealing. Other world cultures, and some Western subcultures, allow more variation in the kinds of female bodies that can be considered sexy. Certainly this is one contributor to the pattern you have noticed. Men who grow up in a culture where there is no encouragement to view bigger women as sexy, and where there are no readily available role models for expressing that attraction, may be less likely to do either one.

Second, we have to look at how race, class, size, and sex create privilege and status, and how racism, classism, sizeism, and sexism support it. In Western culture (and in others as well, such as in East Asian culture) high-class status and thinness go together, and fatness is considered distinctly lower class. At the same time, especially in the West, high-class status also goes along with whiteness. Maleness is also part of high status; men are considered to be higher ranking and more important than women. So whiteness, thinness, and maleness all help to generate higher status and greater privilege. This happens whether a person wants that privilege or intends to have it or not. Privilege and status are a reflection of a culture's values, not of an individual person's desires.

But status can also be lost. And one way to lose status, even for a man with high status, is fatness. And because our sexist society tends to see women as reflections, and possibly possessions, of the men they are with, the fatness need not be his own. Being with a fat woman will lower an otherwise high-status white man's standing. So will admitting to a desire for a woman with a low-status, fat body.

Racism plays into this too. Not to put too fine a point on it, but white men have more status to lose by admitting to a desire for fat partners than men of color do, because white men's whiteness gives them higher status to begin with.

Couple this with mainstream white middle-class culture's ubiquitous, lifelong enculturation of fat-hating and with the difficulty of finding openly fat-attracted role models in white middle-class culture, and there are significant obstacles to white men's free and easy acknowledgment of an attraction to fat people. (Being at the top of the racist, sexist, classist social pyramid of Western culture, which white middle-class men are, whether they want to be or not, exacts its own set of tolls.)

The upshot of all this is that, on the whole, white men probably don't actually desire fat partners any less often than nonwhite men. But they may feel less like they have the latitude to say so, and they may feel that they have more to lose if they do. Whether this is true or not is an open question. In truth it would probably vary, as all such things inevitably do. But the prejudices of the culture remain strong, and so does the fear of what might happen to you if you run afoul of those unwritten rules.

Q: *I don't feel much during penis-in-vagina sex. Is it because my vagina is fat?*

A: No. In fact, the vagina doesn't actually have a whole lot of sensory nerves in it. The majority of the sensory nerves in the female genitalia are packed into the clitoris, not the vagina. If you're not feeling a whole lot of anything when your vagina is penetrated, bear in mind that you actually don't have a whole lot to feel it with. This has to do with the anatomy of the vagina and nothing to do with fat.

Other things that might be affecting how much you feel during vaginal penetration are lubrication; the size of the penis, dildo, or other object that is penetrating you; and to some degree the condition of your pelvic musculature. Whatever vaginal sensation you are going to feel during penis-in-vagina sex happens as a result of friction between the penis and the vaginal walls. Too much lubrication, whether naturally occurring or added by you or your partner, will reduce friction, possibly to the point where you don't feel much. Adding less lubrication, or if need be, removing some of the lubrication your body makes by mopping up with a washcloth, or taking an over-the-counter decongestant (an off-label use, for sure, but it does work for many women) might help if this seems to be the case.

Your partner's penis size may also have something to do with the sensation issue. A small penis may simply not provide much friction against the vaginal walls, particularly if you are built on the wide side. Both penis size and vaginal dimensions are determined by genetics, so what you each have is total luck of the draw. But sometimes a man with a small or slender penis ends up with a woman with a vagina that is naturally on the wider side, which can result in a lack of friction and thus less sensation.

This can be improved to some degree—as can your vaginal sensitivity in general terms—by toning your pelvic musculature with Kegel exercises. To do a Kegel exercise, simply clench your pelvic muscles as if you are cutting off the flow of a stream of urine, hold it for a second or two, then release. Repeating this frequently will help improve the condition of your pelvic musculature, including some of the muscles around the barrel of the vagina, and this in turn may make it possible for you to intentionally create more friction during penetration.

Regardless of what you do, and regardless of the size of your partner's penis, you may still find that vaginal penetration does not provide enough stimulation for you to have an orgasm. Do not despair, and do not assume it's because you're fat: it's actually because you're female and the sensory nerves in your genitals are concentrated in your clitoris. It's hard to get a lot of sensation out of something that doesn't have a lot of sensory nerves. You can't get blood out of a turnip, as my grandmother used to say.

Sticking something into the vagina doesn't necessarily create any friction against the clitoris. Sometimes it can, although it's usually not direct friction but indirect friction. When thrusts into the vagina tug on vulva tissues that are connected to the clitoral hood, the clitoral hood can get tugged on in turn. For some women, this will create a sufficient amount of friction against the clitoris that they will experience an orgasm. But this doesn't happen for all women and may not consistently happen even for women for whom it sometimes works. Statistically, most women do not actually get enough clitoral stimulation from penis-in-vagina intercourse alone to have orgasms. A lot of women simply require more direct and focused stimulation to their clitorises in order to have orgasms. You might be one of them. This is completely normal.

Q: *My belly hangs down and presses my dick down so it's pointing toward the ground even when it's hard. It's hard to get it in and hard to keep it in. What should I do?*

A: You have several options here. The easiest way out is to lie on your back, let everything spread out, and let your partner get on top as you point proudly up to the sky. But maybe you're not feeling like lying back and letting your partner run the fuck, and that's okay too. You might want to try a rear-entry position where you can rest your belly on your partner's tailbone. If your partner is a bit athletic, you could also try a pile-driver position, with your partner's shoulders on the floor, the couch, or the bed and their legs wrapped around your waist so that you penetrate from above. A fourth option is to try sex in the water, because water will help lift up your belly without your having to do anything in particular. Or, if you happen to have a pair of tight-fitting button-fly jeans, try this: a friend reports that if you leave the top two buttons buttoned, and open the bottom two for your junk, the heavy denim can act as traffic control, keeping your belly in one place and preventing your penis from being pushed down. Might be worth a shot.

Q: *I'm embarrassed by the way my fat jiggles when I'm having sex. It makes me feel hideous and I can't get over feeling like my partner secretly thinks so too. How can I jiggle less when I'm having sex?*

A: Honeypie, there are only two things that don't jiggle, bone and silicone. Even at their leanest, human beings are made mostly of water, usually about 60 percent. We are fluid, flowing, jiggling creatures! This means that even the leanest muscle will jiggle a little bit if it's relaxed. Fat jiggles more than muscle, to be sure, but there is nobody—and no body, either—who never jiggles at all.

When it comes to motion, fat has a life of its own. Because the fat that you can see exists immediately under the skin, and doesn't have a lot of connective tissues anchoring it firmly down, it can move around a lot more than, say, your intestines or your kidneys (though even these can move around to some extent). Skin holds it in place, for sure, but skin is flexible. The whole shebang will move around about as far as the skin will allow. Add to that the fact that inertia isn't just a good idea but an actual law—bodies in motion tend to stay in motion until they run out of energy, bodies at rest tend to stay at rest until energy is added—and you understand why fat jiggles and wiggles and joggles and wobbles when you move around. It can't help it. Science!

So the real question here isn't how you can stop jiggling. You can't. Even if you encase yourself in the sturdiest corset known to humankind—and that might be sexy—you're still going to have jiggly bits at either end. Which leaves you where you started, with the problem of getting comfortable in your own skin and with the fact that your wonderful, sexy body is going to jiggle to some extent no matter what you weigh and what you do. As for your partner, don't borrow trouble. Ten'll get you twenty that your partner doesn't have a problem with the way you jiggle. Your partner may even think it's hot (many people do). It's your perception of your own body that is the big problem here, darlin', and the sooner you can learn to accept, or maybe even enjoy, your own jigglitude, the happier your sex life will be.

Resource
Guide

This resource guide is representative, not comprehensive. It does not, and cannot, list absolutely every possible resource that might be of use to fat people and their sexual partners. Listings were chosen based on reputation within the fat-acceptance and sex-positive communities and the responses to the Big Big Love Survey. If we have omitted something of which you are personally fond, as is inevitable in a world with so many options, please accept our apologies.

Listings in this Resource Guide were current and accurate as of the time of publication, but resources can come and go without warning. *Caveat lector.*

General Sex Education and Information

Good Vibrations (www.goodvibes.com). The mothership of feminist sex toy boutiques is also a sex-education clearinghouse, with two PhD sexologists on staff to answer your questions.

Planned Parenthood (www.plannedparenthood.org). Reliable reproductive and sexual health information for all, and local sexual/reproductive health clinics throughout the United States.

San Francisco Sex Information (http://sfsi.org). Volunteer-driven, extremely high-quality free, confidential, accurate, nonjudgmental information about sex and reproductive health online or by phone.

Scarleteen (www.scarleteen.com). Independent and opinionated sex ed website and forums for teens and young adults, but with great info and education for adults of all ages, too.

Boston Women's Health Book Collective. *The New Our Bodies, Our Selves: A Book by and for Women* (New York: Simon and Schuster, 1996).

Cavanah, Claire, and Rachel Venning. *Sex Toys 101: A Playfully Uninhibited Guide* (New York: Simon and Schuster, 2003).

Corinna, Heather. *S.E.X.: The All-You-Need-to-Know Progressive Sexuality Guide to Get You Through High School and College* (New York: Marlowe, 2007).

Newman, Felice. *The Whole Lesbian Sex Book: A Passionate Guide for All of Us* (San Francisco: Cleis Press, 2004).

Seman, Ann, and Cathy Winks. *The Good Vibrations Guide to Sex: The Most Complete Sex Manual Ever Written* (San Francisco: Cleis Press, 2002).

Silverstein, Charles, and Felice Picano. *The Joy of Gay Sex* 3rd ed. (New York: Harper Resource, 2003).

Special Issue Sex Education and Information

Blue, Violet. *The Smart Girl's Guide to Porn* (San Francisco: Cleis Press, 2006).

Dodson, Betty. *Sex for One: The Joy of Selfloving* (New York: Crown Trade Paperbacks, 1996).

Easton, Dossie and Janet W. Hardy. *The Ethical Slut: A Practical Guide to Polyamory, Open Relationships, and Other Adventures* 2nd ed. (Berkeley, CA: Celestial Arts, 2009).

Haines, Staci, and Felice Newman. *Healing Sex: A Mind-Body Approach to Healing Sexual Trauma* (San Francisco: Cleis Press, 2007).

Kaufman, Miriam, Cory Silverberg, and Fran Odette. *The Ultimate Guide to Sex and Disability: For All of Us Who Live With Disabilities, Chronic Pain, and Illness* (San Francisco: Cleis Press, 2003).

Morin, Jack. *Anal Pleasure and Health: A Guide for Men, Women, and Couples* (San Francisco: Down There Press, 2010).

Wiseman, Jay. *SM 101: A Realistic Introduction* (San Francisco: Greenery Press, 1996).

Fat Acceptance and Size Acceptance

Association for Size Diversity and Health (www.sizediversityandhealth .org). Headquartered at Bowling Green State University, ASDAH is an international professional organization composed of individual members who are committed to the Health At Every Size (HAES) principles.

Big Fat Blog (www.bigfatblog.com). A community blog founded in 2000 with a strongly activist size-acceptance focus. Includes news coverage and analysis as well as resources and other discussion.

Council on Size and Weight Discrimination (www.cswd.org). A not-for-profit group that works to change people's attitudes about weight. CSWD acts as a consumer advocate for larger people, especially in the areas of medical treatment, job discrimination, and media images. Mailing Address: CSWD, PO Box 305, Mt. Marion, NY 12456.

International No Diet Day (www.eskimo.com/~largesse/INDD/). Established in 1992, INDD is an annual celebration of body acceptance and diversity. It is celebrated on May 6 each year.

International Size Acceptance Association (www.size-acceptance .org). The ISAA is a voluntary organization with American and international chapters, pursuing issues of size-related advocacy and activism.

They have moved their magazine, *Without Measure*, to blog format at http://womeasure.wordpress.com.

Kelly Bliss' Plus Size Yellow Pages (www.plussizeyellowpages.com). Thousands of size-acceptance resources in a number of categories (organizations, clothing, health/fitness, travel, and so on).

MaryMac's Fat Acceptance Stuff (www.casagordita.com/fatacc.htm). A lovingly curated collection of size-acceptance and fat-friendly resources and links.

National Association for the Advancement of Fat Acceptance (www.naafa.org). Founded in 1969, the National Association to Advance Fat Acceptance (NAAFA) is a nonprofit, all-volunteer, civil rights organization dedicated to protecting the rights of and improving the quality of life for fat people. NAAFA works to eliminate discrimination based on body size and to provide fat people with the tools for self-empowerment through advocacy, public education, and support. Mailing address: NAAFA, Inc. PO Box 22510, Oakland, CA 94609.

Obesity Law and Advocacy Center (www.obesitylaw.com). Established by Walter Lindstrom in 1996, the Obesity Law and Advocacy Center is the first and premier advocacy practice devoted to representing the interests of morbidly obese persons in health care and discrimination matters. Mailing address: 1392 East Palomar Street, Suite 403-233, Chula Vista, CA 91913.

Fraser, Laura. *Losing It: America's Obsession with Weight and the Industry That Feeds on It* (New York: Dutton, 1997).

Harding, Kate, and Marianne Kirby. *Lessons from the Fat-o-sphere: Quit Dieting and Declare a Truce with Your Body* (New York: Perigee Books, 2009).

Oliver, J. Eric. *Fat Politics: The Real Story Behind America's Obesity Epidemic* (New York: Oxford University Press, 2006).

Schwartz, Hillel. *Never Satisfied: A Cultural History of Diets, Fantasies, and Fat* (New York: Free Press, 1986).

Solovay, Sandra. *Tipping the Scales of Justice: Fighting Weight-Based Discrimination* (Amherst, NY: Prometheus Books, 2000).

Solovay, Sandra, and Esther Rothblum, eds. *The Fat Studies Reader* (New York: NYU Press, 2009).

Wann, Marilyn. *Fat!So? Because You Don't Have to Apologize for Your Size* (Berkeley, CA: Ten Speed Press, 1999).

Health and Wellness

Association for Size Diversity and Health (www.sizediversityandhealth .org). Headquartered at Bowling Green State University, ASDAH is an international professional organization composed of individual members who are committed to the Health At Every Size principles.

Body Love Wellness (www.bodylovewellness.com). Golda Poretsky is a consultant and coach specializing in body issues, health, and size acceptance. Based in New York, she provides phone coaching anywhere.

The Fat Friendly Health Professionals List (www.cat-and-dragon.com/ stef/Fat/ffp.html). A regularly updated list of health professionals that have been recommended by fat people as being fat friendly or who have declared themselves fat friendly. The list is arranged alphabetically by country, state, and city.

Plus Size Pregnancy Index (www.plus-size-pregnancy.org). Size-positive, empowering information and resources on plus-sized pregnancies. Exceptionally helpful is its analysis of scientific/medical risk reporting.

Your Plus Size Pregnancy (www.yourplussizepregnancy.com). Information, support, and community for plus-size pregnancies, including an MD-authored e-book on the subject that is officially endorsed by the Department of Gynecology and Obstetrics at the State University of New York at Buffalo School of Medicine and Biomedical Sciences.

Bacon, Linda. *Health at Every Size: The Surprising Truth About Your Weight* (Dallas, TX: BenBella Books, 2008).

Campos, Paul. *The Obesity Myth: Why America's Obsession with Weight Is Hazardous to Your Health* (New York: Gotham Books, 2004).

Gaesser, Glenn. *Big Fat Lies: The Truth About Your Weight and Your Health* (New York: Fawcett Columbine, 1996).

Moser, Charles. *Health Care Without Shame: A Handbook for the Sexually Diverse and Their Caregivers* (San Francisco: Greenery Press, 1999).

Summer, Nancy. *Ample Hygiene for Ample People* (Bearsville, NY: Willendorf Press, N.D.) Note: Available only from Ample Stuff (www.amplestuff.com).

Van der Ziel, Cornelia, and Jacqueline Tourville. *Big, Beautiful, and Pregnant* (New York: Marlowe & Co., 2006).

Hygiene Aids

Amplestuff (www.amplestuff.com). Online retailer of various fat-friendly and fat-focused products, including hygiene tools.

Living XL (www.livingxl.com). Online retailer of fat-friendly products, including a selection of hygiene tools.

Summer, Nancy. *Ample Hygiene for Ample People* (Bearsville, NY: Willendorf Press, N.D.). Note: Available only from Ample Stuff (www.amplestuff.com).

Movement and Injury Prevention

Big Folks Sports and Activities FAQ (www.faqs.org/faqs/fat-acceptance-faq/sports/). An extensive (if somewhat dated) FAQ file giving concrete information and advice about participation in specific sports and activities by fat people.

Big Moves (www.bigmoves.org). Founded in 2000, Big Moves is the only producing, training, and service organization in the world dedicated to getting more people of all sizes into the dance studio and up on stage. Currently operating in California, Massachusetts, New York, and Quebec.

Kelly Bliss (www.kellybliss.com). Kelly Bliss is a lifestyle coach and personal fitness trainer based in Philadelphia who specializes in plus-size fitness and wellness. Kelly's website also has an extensive collection of links and resources.

Living XL (www.livingxl.com). Online shop selling a variety of accessories and equipment for active pursuits including fitness and camping gear geared to the larger/heavier body.

Rochelle Rice (www.infitnessinhealth.com). Rochelle Rice is a personal fitness trainer and the creator of pioneering fitness programs for women of size. Based in New York City.

Anderson, Bob. *Stretching* (Bolinas, CA: Shelter Publications, 2010).

Rice, Rochelle. *Real Fitness for Real Women: A Unique Workout Program for the Plus-Size Woman* (New York: Warner Books, 2001).

Social and Dating Resources

Affiliated Big Men's Clubs (www.abcclubs.com). The Affiliated Big Men's Clubs (ABC) is an umbrella organization for a large number of social organizations focusing on big gay men and their admirers. Includes listings of member clubs and of national and international events relative to fat gay men, including Affiliated Big Men's Clubs' yearly conference.

BBWBelles (www.bbwbelles.com). A popular online destination for big beautiful women (and big handsome men) and their admirers in the American South. BBWBelles also organizes and promotes parties, dinners, picnics, and get-togethers.

BBWclubs (www.bbwclubs.com). A sex-oriented online portal and personals site, mostly heterosexual.

BBW Datefinder (http://bbwdatefinder.com). BBW/FA online personals and chat.

The BBWNetwork (www.bbwnetwork.com). "Our goal is to help promote Size Acceptance and self-esteem. We do not promote gaining weight, we do not promote yo-yo dieting, we do provide an accepting environment no matter what size you are." Sponsors online forums, personal ads, and the yearly Vegas Bash gathering for big women and those who admire them.

Bear411 (www.bear411.com). Online personals for gay male bears.

BearNation Online Community (www.bearnation.us). A major clearinghouse for gay male bears and bear culture, including resources, even listings, blogs, galleries, and personal profiles.

Bulk Male (www.bulkmale.com). Online resources, community, and personal ads for gay chubs and chasers.

Chubby Parade (http://chubbyparade.com). A sex-oriented online portal and personals site, mostly heterosexual.

Chunky Dunk PDX (www.chunkydunkpdx.com). Portland-area swimming parties for fat people and allies. A fabulous idea that would be easy to implement on a DIY basis elsewhere (hint, hint!).

Dimensions (www.dimensionsmagazine.com). The first print magazine to focus on fat women and the men who love them with a size-acceptance perspective, it is now a website that has become a major repository for fat-related news, information, links, resources, and community. Includes forum space specifically for female fat admirers (FFAs), BHMs (Big Handsome Men), and LGBTI fat people and their admirers. The overall focus, however, remains substantially on BBW/FA issues and sexuality, including forums and personals. Note: *Dimensions* is a feederism-accepting space and includes weight-gain and feeding fiction. Extensive discussion of eating and food are also featured in dedicated forum spaces.

Large and Lovely Connections (www.largeandlovely.com). Online personal ads for BBW/FA, and BHM/FFA.

Linda's Big Connections (www.lindasbigconnections.com). A size acceptance group that promotes friendships, relationships, and networking in the BBW/BHM Community in the Chicago/Milwaukee region. Hosts regular parties, dances, and other events.

The Lone Star Saloon (www.lonestarsaloon.com/woof/home). The San Francisco epicenter of the gay male bear world, and the world's first bear bar.

National Organization of Lesbians of Size (www.nolose.org). NOLOSE is "a vibrant community of fat dykes/lesbians, bisexual women, transgendered folks, and allies, seeking to end the oppression of fat people." Hosts an annual conference and sponsors other events in various locations during the year.

Size Acceptance for Empowerment (SAFE) (www.socalsafe.org). Size Acceptance for Empowerment offers a place where men and women of all sizes can enjoy a size-friendly atmosphere. Activism focuses around social events, with an active calendar.

Transgender People of Size (http://tgpos.livejournal.com). A participatory online community for transgender people of size, on the popular LiveJournal journal hosting site.

Size-Positive Imagery, Erotica, and Pornography

Adipositivity (http://adipositivity.com). Photographer Substantia Jones's size-acceptance activism takes the form of a lush, beautifully crafted photoblog of her artistic nudes and other photos of women of all sizes of large.

April Flores (www.fattyd.com). The undisputed current queen of BBW erotic modeling and pornography, April Flores is also an artist's muse and a genial blogger.

Bear (www.bear-magazine.com). Founded in 1987, "the original periodical specifically geared toward gay men who are or who admire real masculine men, proudly sporting body and facial hair" is now back in publication.

Bulk Male (www.bulkmale.com). Gay male chub/chaser portal, personals, galleries, and more.

Fat Bottom Boudoir (www.fatbottomboudoir.com). Seattle-based photographer Molly Bennett's size-positive boudoir photography, including extensive galleries.

Men in Full (http://men-in-full.tumblr.com). Images of fat men, presented by a woman who loves them.

The Museum of Fat Love (http://love.twowholecakes.org). A museum of photos of fat people in love, many with personal narratives. Guaranteed to bring a smile to your face.

Nofauxxx (www.nofauxxx.com). Award-winning pornographer Courtney Trouble's wonderfully diverse porn site, featuring performers of all genders, sizes, skin colors, and sexual orientations.

The Sex Positive Photo Project (http://thesexpositivephotoproject.blogspot .com). Photographer Shilo McCabe's adventurous, sex-positive, size-inclusive photoblog.

The Thickness (http://thethickness.tumblr.com). A regularly updated Tumblr feed of erotic/pornographic photos of curvy/thick/fat women.

Toil Girls (www.toilgirls.com). Home of the BBW pinup artist Les Toil, with galleries and information on how you or someone you love can be rendered as a Toil Girl.

Blank, Hanne, ed. *Zaftig: Well Rounded Erotica* (San Francisco: Cleis Press, 2001).

Edison, Laurie Toby, and Debbie Notkin. *Women En Large: Images of Fat Nudes* (San Francisco: Books in Focus, 1994).

Nimoy, Leonard. *The Full Body Project: Photographs by Leonard Nimoy* (New York: Five Ties, 2007).

Olson, Nancy. *This Is Who I Am: Our Beauty in All Shapes and Sizes* (New York: Artisan, 2008).

St. Paige, Edward. *Zaftig: The Case for Curves.* (Seattle, WA: Darling & Co., Blue Lantern Studio, 1999).

Suresha, Ron Jackson, ed. *Bearotica: Hot, Hairy, Heavy Fiction* (Los Angeles: Alyson Books, 2002).

Sex Toys and Accessories

While not all toys and accessories will work for, or even appeal to, all people, the items listed below have earned a reputation among sex-positive fat folks as among the most useful, reliable, and fat friendly.

Crown dildo harness by Stormy Leather (stormyleather.com). Designed for fuller figures, with a wider hip band, intended to be worn higher than other harnesses. Fits up to a 40-inch waist and 60-inch hip.

Divine Diva dildo harness by Sportsheets (www.sportsheets.com). One of the most adjustable dildo harnesses, can fit up to an 82-inch waist.

Eroscillator (http://eroscillator.com). Primarily an external/clitoral vibrator, with multiple attachments and a long handle.

Fleshlight (www.fleshlight.com). Masturbation sleeve for people with penises, with a rigid, lengthy casing, available with many different options.

Flex-o-Pleaser vibrator. Made by California Exotics, an oval-shaped vibrating head on the end of a long, flexible wand, with an additional handle. Excellent for reach.

Hitachi Magic Wand Massager. Extremely popular long-handled powerful plug-in massager that can be used as an external/clitoral vibrator, attachments available for internal use.

Joque dildo harness by SpareParts Hardwear (sparepartshardwear.com). Recommended by many survey respondents. In size B, fits waists from 35 to 65 inches.

Liberator Sex Shapes and Sex Furniture (www.liberator.com). Purpose-built sex supports and furniture with easily cleanable covers. Amply sized and sturdy. Factory store is in Atlanta.

Sex Sling by Sportsheets (www.sportsheets.com). A long, adjustable webbing strap with leg cuffs at either end and a padded collar in the middle, designed to pass behind the neck and shoulders to hold the legs up with less effort.

Wahl Massager. A popular long-handled, powerful plug-in massager that can be used as an excellent external/clitoral vibrator.

Fat-Friendly Sex Toy and Accessories Vendors

These vendors and businesses are among those known to be fat friendly. Other vendors may be fat friendly as well, but these have excellent track records.

Babeland (www.babeland.com). Brick-and-mortar stores in Seattle and New York, woman owned. In business since 1993.

Blowfish (www.blowfish.com). Online-only store, in business since 1994, with extensive and knowledgeable product reviews.

Come as You Are (www.comeasyouare.com). Cooperatively worker-owned Toronto store in business since 1997. Has exceptional sex and disability resources.

Early to Bed (www.early2bed.com). Woman-owned Chicago shop, in business since 2001.

Good for Her (www.goodforher.com). Woman-owned Toronto shop, in business over eleven years. Physical store features women and trans-only shopping hours.

Good Vibrations (www.goodvibes.com). The grandmother of all feminist sex-toy stores, founded in 1977, has physical stores in the San Francisco area and in Brookline, Massachusetts.

Love U (www.loveuparties.com). Woman-run sex toy party company; individual consultants are well trained and products are carefully chosen.

Self Serve (www.selfservetoys.com). A woman-owned shop in Albuquerque with an emphasis on education and empowerment.

Smitten Kitten (www.smittenkitten.com). Minneapolis' women-owned, ethically sound sex boutique. A second shop is in Denver.

Stockroom (www.stockroom.com). Sex gear of all kinds with a focus on BDSM, with a physical store in Los Angeles and online store, since 1988.

Sugar (www.sugartheshop.com). Since 2007, Baltimore's woman-owned, socially conscious sex boutique.

Womyn's Ware (www.womynsware.com). In business since 1995, this woman-owned shop is located online and in Vancouver.

Lingerie and Clothing

About Curves (www.aboutcurves.com). Online vendor of pretty, feminine women's lingerie including bridal and peignoir sets, to 7X.

Big Gals Lingerie (www.biggalslingerie.com). Online vendor of off-the-rack (to 6X) and custom (to 12X) women's lingerie, club wear, swimwear, and more.

Dark Garden (www.darkgarden.com). Superb off-the-rack and custom corsetry for all sexes and genders, based in San Francisco. Pricey but phenomenal.

Frederick's of Hollywood (www.fredericksofhollywood.com). A wide range of classic women's lingerie and undergarments to size 3X.

FTM at Underworks (http://ftm.underworks.com). Breast binders and related shape wear for FTMs, butches, and others who want to create or enhance a masculine shape. Most items to a 3X, some to a 6X.

Hips and Curves (www.hipsandcurves.com). Online vendor of off-the-rack (to 6x) women's lingerie, corsets, and other things.

Mr. S/Madame S. (www.mr-s-leather.com). Comprehensive selection of leather and fetish gear extending well beyond clothes, but the clothes in some cases do go up past the "regular" size range.

Re/Dress NYC (www.redressnyc.com). Revolutionary plus-size vintage and consignment in Brooklyn, NY, served up in a 3,000-square-foot shop with plenty of sass, fun, and glamour. If you're in New York, go.

Sanctuaire (www.sanctuarie.net). Online vendor of off-the-rack women's clothing and lingerie, including Halloween costumes, to 9x.

Size Queen Clothing (www.bigboxers.com). Portland-based designer Bertha Pearl's feisty, fun indie designs including boxers for both men and women, bloomers, club wear, hot pants, and more to 8x.

Stormy Leather (www.stormyleather.com). San Francisco's legendary leather, fetishwear, and sexual accessories manufacturer. A wide range of sizes in garments and accessories for people of all sexes and genders.

Torrid (www.torrid.com). Nationwide chain of trendy plus-size shops for women, also offering online sales. Good for sexy street wear and club wear at affordable prices, although you should be aware that quality varies.

About the Author

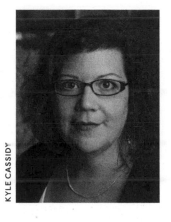

KYLE CASSIDY

Hanne Blank is a writer and historian. Her work has been featured in *Penthouse, In These Times, Southwest Art, Lilith, Bitch: Feminist Response to Pop Culture*, the *Baltimore CityPaper*, the *Boston Phoenix, Santa Fean Magazine*, and others. Her short fiction and essays are frequently anthologized. Hanne's work has been reviewed in the *New York Times*, the *Chicago Sun-Times*, the *Washington Post*, the *Village Voice, NYLON, Entertainment Weekly*, and many other periodicals, and she has been widely interviewed on radio and television in the United States, Australia, United Kingdom, and Canada, including being featured on National Public Radio, BBC 4, and on the acclaimed Canadian program SexTV. As a public speaker and educator, Hanne has appeared on the campuses of many universities and colleges, as well as at national and regional conferences of various types and centers for adult learning. She has taught at the university level at Brandeis University, Tufts University, and Whitworth College. Formally trained as a classical musician, Hanne currently lives and works in Baltimore, Maryland, where she shares a 170-year-old stone house on a dirt road in the middle of the city with her spouse, two cats, and the world's cutest Japanese Akita. Find her online at www.hanneblank.com.

Index

Boundaries, creating and enforcing,
    21–25, 125, 126
Breasts, enlargement of, 157–58
Bulk Male, 211, 212

C
Chairs, 29, 30–31
Chubby Parade, 211
Chub chasers, 7, 61
Chubs, 61–62
Chunky Dunk PDX, 211
Cleanliness, 16–17, 40–44
Cleis Press, 179
Clitoris, stimulation of, 199,
    200–201
Clothing
    as armor, 91, 92
    choosing, 36–40, 76
    sources of, 216
Come as You Are, 215
Compliments, 86–87
Consent, enthusiastic, 68, 158–62
Contraception, 136–37
Cosmetics, 41
Council on Size and Weight
    Discrimination (CSWD), 206
Cunnilingus. See Oral sex
Cushions, 163, 164

D
Dark Garden, 216
Dating
    family and, 105–7
    resources, 210–12
Desire, loss of, 47–49, 144–45
Desperation, sexual, 8–9
Dieting, 47–49
Dildo harnesses, 181–83, 214
Dildos, 168, 169, 180, 183
Dimensions magazine, 178, 211
Discipline. See BDSM

Doctors
    choosing, 149
    visiting, 148–52
Doggy style, 172–73
Dominance. See BDSM
Dyspareunia, 146–47

E
Early to Bed, 215
Erectile dysfunction, 145–46
Erotica, 177–79, 212–13
Exercise, 49–52, 142

F
Face sitting, 184–85
Faking it, 73, 79–80
Family
    dealing with, 101–3, 104–6
    supportive, 106–7
Fashion, 36–40
Fat
    as fetish, 189–92
    jiggling, 202
    rearranging, for sex, 165
    use of word, 3
Fat acceptance/size acceptance, 26, 60,
    62–63, 94, 194, 206–8
Fat admirers (FAs)
    coming out, 114, 115–22
    definition of, 6, 56
    diversity of, 56–57, 112, 113–14
    ethics and, 122–27
    ethnicities of, 197–99
    gay, 61–62
    harassment of, 116–17, 119
    issues faced by, 57–58, 115–22
    mainstream views of, 115–17
    number of, 112–13
    political/social support from, 120,
        127–31
    porn for, 177–79
    subculture of, 7

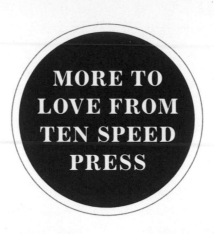
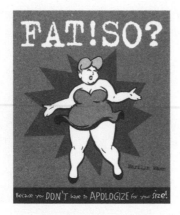
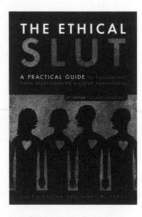